Praise for
Growing Up Healthy

"In *Growing Up Healthy,* former *Good Morning America* host Joan Lunden and pediatrician Myron Winick team up to help parents raise children with healthy eating habits. They start with pregnancy and move through each developmental stage, addressing questions about which foods are healthiest, how to handle finicky eaters and how to deal with the American love affair with food."

—*The Daily News of Los Angeles*

"[This book] teaches parents how to feed their children from the womb through adolescence, how to teach their children good health and eating habits and how to add quality years to their children's life."

—*Chicago Daily Herald*

"In light of recent medical news—that poor diet and inactivity may overtake tobacco as the #1 cause of preventable death in America—Joan Lunden's new book is especially timely."

—*Ladies Home Journal*

"Heart disease, diabetes, hypertension can begin in childhood. *Growing Up Healthy* by former *Good Morning America* co-host Joan Lunden and Dr. Myron Winick prescribes a nutrition plan that begins in the womb."

—*Publishers Weekly*

"All parents want their kids to enjoy good health. And Joan, who has three daughters . . . and two twins, is no different. Now, thanks to her work with Dr. Winick, their book . . . will give other parents the information they need to help their children grow up healthy."

—*National Enquirer*

Also by Joan Lunden

Healthy Living

Healthy Cooking

A Bend in the Road

Wake-Up Calls

Good Morning, I'm Joan Lunden

Joan Lunden Mothers' Minutes

Also by Dr. Myron Winick

The Fiber Prescription

Hunger Disease

Nutrition, Pregnancy and Early Infancy

Your Personalized Health Profile: Choosing the Diet That's Right for You

Malnutrition and Brain Development

Dr. Myron Winick's Growing Up Healthy: Parent's Guide to Good Nutrition

For Mothers & Daughters: A Guide to Good Nutrition for Women

Nutrition in Health and Disease

Nutrition and Pregnancy

Growing Up Healthy

A Complete Guide to Childhood
Nutrition, Birth Through Adolescence

JOAN LUNDEN and
MYRON WINICK, MD

ATRIA BOOKS

New York   London   Toronto   Sydney

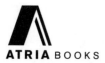

ATRIA BOOKS

1230 Avenue of the Americas
New York, NY 10020

Photo credits: p. 11, 77 © ABC-TV/Ida Mae Astute; p. 63 © Jacques Silberstein; p. 72 Reprinted with permission © 2003 American Lung Association. For more information on how you can support to fight lung disease, the third leading cause of death in the U.S., please contact the American Lung Association at 1-800-LUNG-USA (1-800-586-4872) or visit the website at www.lungusa.org http://www.lungusa.org; p. 75 Larry Busacca, Wire Image; p. 114 Gina Coleman; p. 120 © New Life Entertainment/Tom Eckerle; p. 134 © Timothy White; p. 145 © 1995 National Fluid Milk Processor Promotion Board; p. 189 Nicole Bril; photos on pp. 20, 40, 43, 49, 83, 89, 97, 113, 160, 180 from the personal collection of Joan Lunden; photos on pp. 3, 69, 190, 202 from the personal collection of Dr. Myron Winick.

Designed by Joel Avirom and Jason Snyder

ISBN-13: 978-0-7434-8614-9
         978-0-7434-8368-1 (Pbk)
ISBN-10:   0-7434-8614-5
           0-7434-8368-5 (Pbk)

First Atria Books trade paperback edition July 2005

10 9 8 7 6 5 4 3 2 1

ATRIA BOOKS is a trademark of Simon & Schuster, Inc.

Manufactured in the United States of America

For information regarding special discounts for bulk purchases, please contact Simon & Schuster Special Sales at 1-800-456-6798 or business@simonandschuster.com

This book became a reality because, from the very beginning days of his career as a pediatrician, Dr. Myron Winick recognized the important relationship between childhood nutrition and adult, chronic disease. He always felt in his heart of hearts that he and his colleagues should be doing more than just inoculating their little patients against diseases. His theories, linking nutrition and disease, were validated when he got the much needed backing from the American Health Foundation, who appointed him to lead the task force to study that link. Children everywhere will benefit from Dr. Winick's strong convictions, and the relentless research and critical support of all the medical professionals involved.

Joan Lunden

To Elaine and to my grandson Bradley, who I hope will grow up strong and healthy.

Myron Winick

Contents

Acknowledgments

(*Joan Lunden*)

I thought it best to begin with my new twins, Kate and Max, since their impending birth was my biggest motivation for this valuable project. I feel fortunate to have been given this opportunity to educate myself so thoroughly on how I can protect them from chronic disease and help them live long, healthy lives. I would also like to acknowledge my surrogate, Deborah Bolig, who gave Kate and Max their start at life—you and Pete and your daughters Alexandra, Victoria, and Kate will always be part of our family.

At times writing this book actually reminded me of how it feels to be pregnant! The writing process can give you the munchies and keep you up all night. You create new parts every day, and you *definitely* need the support of a devoted family. You might say it's a "labor-intensive" project that involves all of your loved ones. To my loving husband, Jeff, and my five amazing children, Jamie, Lindsay, Sarah, Kate, and Max, I thank you all for putting up with the never-ending writing sessions, and especially the all-nighters that were necessary to produce a book like this. Not to mention your patience for allowing me to try out my recipes on you. Thanks to your unforgiving taste buds, not all of the possible recipes ended up in the final manuscript.

While this book is the brainchild of Dr. Myron Winick, there are a number of other health professionals who contributed so much. My most sincere appreciation goes to pediatric and adolescent nutritionist Michelle Daum (a mom of three), who is in private practice in Westchester and Long Island, New York. She dedicated a considerable amount of time and attention to ensure that we got everything right. Also generous with her time, not to mention her hands-on expertise in caring for children, was Dr. Lauren Carton, a Westchester pediatrician who is also a mother of two. Liz Shaio is a clinical nutritionist who works with young children and adolescents, and worked with us as well, offering much needed practical advice. Liz is associated with the Wilkins Center in Greenwich, Connecticut. That center was founded by Dr. Diane Mickley, an internist who specializes in eating disorders, and who also contributed her time and expertise for this book. Mary Beth Augustine is a medical nutrition therapist with the Continuum Center for Health and Healing at Beth Israel Hospital in New York City, and a mother of two. A cancer survivor, she feels strongly that we can prevent disease and slow down its growth through nutrition. She urges mothers to start thinking about protecting their children through diet, beginning in the womb. Executive chef Leora Perlman, new mom and cofounder of Diva's Delite Catering & Opera in New York City, fine-tuned our recipes so they would be delicious as well as nutritious. And finally, fitness trainer and mother of two, Beth Bielat, was our exercise consultant. We thank her for her advice on how to better motivate and inspire children to be physically active, so that they will grow up with healthier lifelong habits.

When it came time to compile our healthy, kid-friendly recipes, I turned to some wonderful restaurants. Sal Scognamilo, who owns Patsy's restaurant, at 236 West 56th Street in New York City, always took special care in preparing foods that my girls would enjoy. I was so excited when he offered to share a few of those recipes with our readers. And many thanks go to Sirio Maccioni and his lovely wife, Egi, who own the world-famous Le Cirque restaurant, and who were kind enough to share recipes from their latest cookbook, *The Maccioni Family Cookbook*. Lisa Vitielo, who owns DaVinci's restaurant on Greenwich Avenue, in Greenwich, Connecticut, loves to cook for her patrons, her children, and her grandchildren. She dove into her personal recipe file looking for just the right dishes for our readers. Sergio Brasesco took the reins from his father, who founded Emilio's restaurant on Colonial Place in Harrison, New York, and has continued the tradition of excellent service and superb food. We thank him for creating several original recipes for us. Route 22 in Armonk, New York, is the brainchild of Lance Root. The restaurant caters to kids and families in both its décor and its menu. We're thrilled that he shared some of his kid-friendly recipes with us. And of course my good buddy, Wolfgang Puck, is always there for me whenever I ask for some good recipes to share, and this was no exception. I've learned a lot about cooking from Wolfgang's many visits to the *Good Morning America* set, and I think your family will enjoy his yummy contributions. And finally a special thanks to Susan Westmoreland and all the folks at the *Good Housekeeping* Test Kitchen for the recipes they shared with us, as well as all their assistance throughout the writing of the book.

We were fortunate to have two wonderful writers working with us on this project, Gail North and Janet Roth. They relentlessly tracked down research, and brilliantly blended together the work of Dr. Winick and the task force together with my personal experience, in order to help create a mommy-friendly guide that would be helpful to parents and children everywhere.

A trusted friend and my literary agent for ten years now, Al Lowman was there for me as always, throughout the writing of this book to help guide me and inspire me. My sincerest thanks for his selfless efforts in the editing, book design, and publicity and promotion of this project. I am lucky to have someone like Al in my life, someone with such incredible literary instincts and someone who always knows how to bring out the best in me.

Of course the book would not have been possible without the support of our publisher, Judith Curr, who truly has a desire to help parents everywhere raise healthy children. My deep appreciation also goes to my relentless editor, Brenda Copeland, who worked so incredibly hard to make the writing process much more enjoyable and our words so much more succinct. Thanks also to her tireless assistant, Samantha Martin. Paolo Pepe, John Paul Jones, Jamie Putorti, and the entire art and production team at Atria did a wonderful job making the book enjoyable to read, inside and out. The publicity team headed up by Seale Ballenger was outstanding in plotting an effective promotional campaign to spread the word to parents everywhere about these important medical findings. And thanks also go to Ellen Geiger, the agent on this project who was able to bring all of us together to make this book possible.

A special thank you goes to Melinda Kristofich who took time out from running my production company to obtain the photo rights to every picture in this book, and coordinate every detail with all of the health professionals and chefs who so kindly shared their recipes with us.

I am also grateful to the very talented photographer Andrew Eccles, who shot the photograph on the cover of this book. We have worked together many times over the years on various magazine covers and when I needed his assistance to use the cover photo, he made it happen. A new dad himself, he made a very wiggly photo session with my newborn twins an absolute delight.

Acknowledgments

(Dr. Winick)

Thanks to my wife, Elaine, always my first editor, and to my brother, Dr. Paul Winick, my favorite pediatrician, for his practical advice. Thanks also to my agent, Ellen Geiger, for all her help.

A Pediatrician's Passionate Plea to Parents

By Dr. Myron Winick

When I was a young pediatrician, the guiding principle of my profession was to ensure proper growth and development in children. Unlike other medical specialists, however, we pediatricians also had a particular interest in prevention. We made sure that children were vaccinated against smallpox, diphtheria, tetanus, and whooping cough, diseases that had caused misery and death. Over the last thirty years, other vaccines became available, and we were able to prevent diseases like polio, measles, mumps, chickenpox, hepatitis, and others. All of this, in addition to treating sick children. Not much has changed in that area, and this approach is still valid.

Today, however, we look at disease prevention not only as immunizing children against infectious diseases, but also as reducing the risk for certain chronic diseases found almost exclusively in adults. A whole new era in the care of children is beginning, the era of focusing on what researchers call pediatric antecedents of adult disease—the link between childhood nutrition and chronic illness in later years.

We now know that many of the symptoms of disease associated with adulthood make their first appearance in childhood—and it is in childhood that steps need to be taken to effectively diagnose, treat, and possibly prevent these diseases.

Our new, groundbreaking research shows that many of the diseases we all associate with old age—heart disease, stroke, osteoporosis, hypertension, cancer, and diabetes—actually begin during childhood, and that poor nutrition and the development of unhealthy eating habits take their toll later in life. We now know that early stages of many of these chronic diseases can be detected in children. Decades of painstaking research and testing have shown that the buildup of plaque deposits in arteries, just to cite an example, is apparent in young people who are consuming a typical American diet loaded with fat. Feeding children right in the years when their young bodies are growing and organs and tissues are developing is the best way to shield them from many of the diseases that won't show up as symptoms until much later in life.

How does nutrition in children play a role in preventing some of the most serious chronic diseases seen in adults? If we have learned anything in the last few years, we have learned that the major killer diseases that plague Western society are caused by many factors, and in most of these diseases nutrition is a major factor. Most Americans will die of cardiovascular disease, stroke, or cancer. Millions of Americans will have to learn to live with diabetes, high blood pressure, and osteoporosis. All of these diseases develop at least in part because of poor nutrition—excesses or deficiencies—too much of one thing or not enough of another. We now recognize that because of the diets our children consume, some of these diseases may begin in early childhood or infancy— even in the womb. *More importantly, we now know that our intervention can affect the progress of those diseases and perhaps change the course of our children's lives.*

Nutrition in infants and children has been my major interest for all of my professional life. For more than thirty years, I've been a pediatrician and a professor of pediatrics and nutrition. My research has focused on nutrition and growth, particularly the growth of the brain, as well as the effects of undernutrition on physical growth and mental development. Over the years, I've maintained my suspicion that a direct link between childhood nutrition and adult disease does exist. Four years ago, I became chairman of a task force for The American Health Foundation, overseeing and compiling studies for a program aimed at preventing adult disease through childhood nutrition. The findings from this literature have validated my suspicion—and they are nothing short of remarkable.

The discovery of this critical link affects everyone across all socioeconomic lines, from the most affluent of families to the poorest. Affluence does not ensure long life. Even parents in the most privileged circumstances can be unwittingly feeding their children foods that will increase their risk for malnutrition and chronic disease in their adult years.

Prior to the discovery of the link between childhood nutrition and adult disease, most of us had little idea of how important the food we provided our children could be to their future health. Now we know. The foods we place on our children's plates, in their lunch boxes, and in their snacks can make a major difference. Beginning with pregnancy, feeding them the right foods can give them the best shot at living healthier, and very probably longer lives.

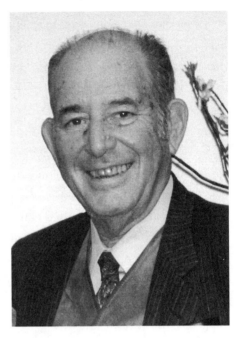

Dr. Myron Winick. A pioneer in the field of childhood health and nutrition.

To better understand how most of the important diseases that afflict older Americans may begin in childhood, you need look no further than obesity. Obesity is a major factor for high blood pressure and Type II diabetes, each of which by itself is a major risk factor for heart disease and stroke. In addition, obesity increases a person's risk for certain cancers, for gallbladder disease, and for the complications of any type of surgery. So if we could prevent an adult from being obese or prevent a child from becoming an obese adult, we would improve the adult's health greatly.

We now know that a child who is obese at age four has a greater than 80 percent chance of becoming an obese adult if nothing is done to prevent it. Childhood obesity is a very special kind of obesity. Studies have found that it's much more difficult to treat obese adults who were obese as children than obesity that develops after childhood. It stands to reason then that if we wish to prevent the complications of obesity in many adults, we must prevent it from occurring during childhood. And if it hasn't been treated in early childhood, we must take action and begin to treat it immediately.

3

Not only is obesity striking at an earlier age, but we're also seeing the beginnings of heart disease earlier in children. The sad fact is that more Americans will die of heart disease than any other illness. Heart disease begins when a thin whitish streak of fat is deposited in the arterial wall. These streaks are now showing up in children as young as ten.

We first noticed these fatty streaks in 60 percent of our young soldiers who died of wounds received in the Korean and Vietnam wars. By contrast, almost none of the Korean or Vietnamese soldiers who died of wounds showed these streaks. What we learned from this is that by the time our young sons are in their late teens or early twenties, a majority of them already show signs of coronary heart disease. Why? The American diet contains too much dietary fat, particularly saturated fat, and too much cholesterol, which are all directly related to coronary artery disease.

Iron is a nutrient that further complicates the heart picture. Recent findings demonstrate that large accumulations of iron increase the risk of coronary heart disease, especially in boys. These findings have caused us to reevaluate who should receive iron supplements during later childhood, when, how much, and whether the practice of supplementation should be different for boys and girls. This is something that should be discussed with your doctor.

Another nutrient consumed in excess that contributes to serious heart disease is salt (sodium). When consumed in excess, salt increases our children's risk for high blood pressure, a condition that leads to hypertension and eventually can lead to coronary heart disease. Our children are not born with a taste for salt. It's a learned, acquired taste.

Unlike salt, a liking for the sweet taste of sugar is inborn. Sugar (particularly in a gummy or sticky form) is very dangerous to developing teeth and must be consumed by children in moderation. It is also a source of empty calories. Consuming too much sugar may deprive a child of other important nutrients, nutrients that may lower the risk for cancer and increase the risk factor for serious vitamin and mineral deficiencies.

While we want to avoid an excess of sodium and iron, there are nutrients for which the reverse is true. Calcium is the best example. Here, the adult disease we hope to nip in the bud is osteoporosis. This is a disease in which progressive bone loss, particularly in women after menopause, can result in fractures of the vertebrae, hips, and extremities. Bone growth begins in the womb and continues throughout childhood and, in fact, is active throughout adolescence. Calcium is the key to bone growth. During our children's growth years, calcium must be available in sufficient amounts and in the proper form.

Important changes in our children's diets and eating patterns can also lessen their risk for cancer. We know that certain types of diets offer protection against various cancers and that the longer these diets are consumed the greater the protection. Rather than consuming more or less of a simple nutrient, protection from cancer requires altering our children's dietary patterns.

I believe that it is vitally important for parents to encourage an anticancer food plan for our children. The recommended food plan is low in fat, high in dietary fiber, loaded with vitamins all found in fruits and vegetables, and contains only sufficient calories to maintain ideal weight.

I hope by now you understand that we have it within our power to protect our children from some of the most devastating diseases of old age. And I hope you understand that by feeding our children the right foods and helping them to develop healthy eating patterns, we offer them the most precious of gifts—the best chance for a long life, free of disease. It does take resolve, but by taking control of our children's future health now, it's not hard to imagine them enjoying life for six, seven, or even eight decades down the road. I call this new resolve, love.

And that is what my passionate plea to parents is all about. I'm asking all of you to take this information seriously. The link between childhood nutrition and adult disease is real, and the findings here are critically important to your entire family.

Finally, of all the writing projects with which I've been involved that deal with nutrition in general and nutrition in children specifically, I am most excited by the information contained in *Growing Up Healthy.* However, I am quite aware that these critical research findings won't alter the course of our children's lives unless someone who has actually made a difference for parents steps up to share them with you.

For that reason, I teamed up with one of America's most famous and visible working moms, Joan Lunden. A passionate advocate for parents and children over the years, Joan has distinguished herself as a respected and eloquent communicator. During her many years as a host on *Good Morning America,* she eagerly brought parenting issues into our homes and made them easy to understand. She not only shared important and often intimate information concerning her personal experience as a mother, but also easily assimilated and interpreted new findings from parenting professionals.

I had the good fortune of appearing on *Good Morning America* with Joan many times—and it was a pleasure. As she interviewed me on topics regarding children's health, I was impressed with her questions and her facility for demystifying complicated medical issues—and I still am. Joan does her homework. In this book, she couples her abiding respect for science with her profound love for children—and she does it using language all parents will understand. We make a great team.

I'm extremely pleased and proud that Joan has partnered with me to share this invaluable, breakthrough guide with you.

Myron Winick, MD

PART I

The Remarkable Link Between Childhood Nutrition and Adult Diseases

1

Killer Diseases Begin with Childhood Nutrition

I'm a new mom all over again! And just as excited and in awe of the challenge of parenthood as I was first time around. My new twins now have an amazing opportunity to live longer, healthier lives, free of chronic disease. When I was raising Jamie, Lindsay, and Sarah, my three older daughters, I was constantly sifting through books and magazines in search of trustworthy pediatric health news, as I'm sure you are. Throughout my years as cohost on *Good Morning America,* parenting and the importance of sound childhood nutrition were subjects about which I was always passionate.

Now that my husband Jeff and I have been blessed with our amazing twins, I'm

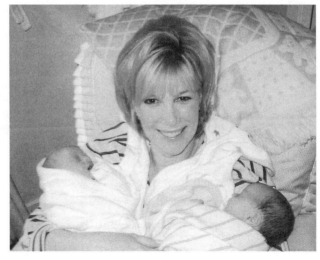

Double the joy second time around!

reminded that raising a child into a healthy, happy, and productive adult is one of the most rewarding things a person can do—and one of the most daunting. So, once again, I found myself searching for the latest findings on how to give a child the healthiest life possible. That's when I was introduced to renowed pediatric nutritionist Dr. Myron Winick, who headed up one of the most important studies in the area of childhood health and nutrition. The three-year task force commissioned by the American Health Foundation produced what just might be the most important medical breakthrough to come along in years: the definitive link between childhood nutrition and chronic illness in later life.

Dr. Winick contacted me to see if I would be interested in helping to get this vitally important news out to other parents. I had first met Dr. Winick in 1984 when I interviewed him on *Good Morning America* for his earlier book on feeding children, also entitled *Growing Up Healthy*. Those of us at *Good Morning America* found him to be such an effective communicator of this type of practical parenting advice that we invited him back on the program regularly. One of our country's leading experts in the field of pediatric nutrition, Dr. Winick later spearheaded the study to examine the significance of our children's diets on chronic illness. The task force findings showed that we as parents have it within our power to help protect our children from disease and very possibly lengthen their lives.

As a concerned parent, I feel privileged to pass along this information to parents everywhere. I think you will agree that it contains some of the most important health and nutritional findings to emerge in decades.

If you're like me, you too love your kids passionately and are eager to learn the secret to possibly lengthening their lives. You want them to be free from the killer diseases plaguing our society; you want them to be happy and blossom into strong, healthy adults; you want them to stay vigorous and fit into their nineties. (Did I say nineties? How about imagining our children as healthy centenarians!) Very simply, you don't want them to get sick! What you do want is to learn how to take control of their nutrition and give them the gift of a life infused with good health.

I know that you work hard, that you're probably pooped out, stressed out, and barraged with the latest information about what you should and shouldn't do for the care and feeding of your children—and who to trust. Believe me, I know, I'm right there with you. That's why I feel so lucky to have found Dr. Winick's research on nutrition, so as to better understand this link between our children's diets and adult disease. I feel that I'm arming myself with this life-saving knowledge to help shield my children from illness and to help them grow into strong, fit adults.

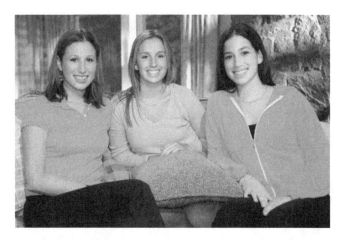

Big sisters Jamie, Lindsay, and Sarah.

Over the past year while I've been working on this book with Dr. Winick, I've had the opportunity to share much of this groundbreaking information with my older girls, Jamie, Lindsay, and Sarah. I can already see what a wonderfully healthy influence it's having on their behaviors. Which reminds me, that just as it's never too early to introduce healthy habits, it's never too late.

Like so many of us, I didn't learn my own personal nutrition lessons until somewhat later in life. While I always understood that my children needed a good foundation for growth and development, quite frankly, I didn't have one myself. It wasn't until I was almost forty that I started paying closer attention to my own fitness and nutrition and launched my own health odyssey. Actually, it was the constant interviews with health experts on the morning show that prompted me to wake up and get serious about my health. And so, I began an exercise program; I changed the way I ate; I lost fifty pounds; and I probably added twenty years to my life. I'd like to see children everywhere add years to their lives, too.

That's why I've come on board to be the voice for this exciting project: I want parents everywhere to become recipients of this most loving gift—an opportunity to give our children the best shot at growing up healthy and circumventing adult diseases.

This information is critically important for every family. By paying careful attention to the foods we're popping into our children's mouths and making some important alterations in their diets, we can become *take-action parents* on the front lines of defense against future illness. I look at this as disease intervention.

Training our children to become conscious of their food choices is part of that intervention. I would venture to say that teaching our children sound eating guidelines is equally as important as teaching them about Mesopotamia. Doesn't it seem logical that both history *and* nutrition are crucial to a complete education?

Our children begin to develop food preferences in early infancy that will remain with them throughout their lives. When we as parents begin to understand this on a gut level, we'll want to maximize their odds by helping them to develop a friendly, positive relationship with healthy foods.

Quite frankly, when I first heard about the direct link between childhood nutrition and adult disease, I was flabbergasted. I began to read as many reports as I could about this important link and found that the implications were staggering. Here are two samples from the U.S. government:

- The U.S. Department of Health and Human Services reports that unhealthy eating and inactivity cause 310,000 to 580,000 deaths every year—similar to the number of deaths caused by tobacco; thirteen times more than are caused by guns; and twenty times more than by drug use!

- The U.S. Surgeon General's Report on Nutrition and Health tells us that two-thirds of all deaths are related to what we eat. This includes deaths from heart disease, stroke, diabetes, osteoporosis, and cancer. The report highlights that many of the diet-associated chronic diseases of adulthood begin in childhood.

While we should all find these reports alarming, I think it's important that we also view them as motivating. And this is where we, as parents, come in. To understand the necessity of early intervention, let's take a look at how childhood nutrition links to obesity, the development of heart disease and stroke, high blood pressure, Type II diabetes, cancer, and osteoporosis.

Obesity—Much More Than Just a Weight Problem

We only have to watch kids in school yards (no matter how oversize their pants!), or listen to the nightly news to understand how prevalent obesity has become in our society. Yet, while we're aware of this growing epidemic, much of our focus has been on *thinness*. Children can be cruel, and none of us want our sons and daughters to be ridiculed because they're fat. But our preoccupation with looking good misses the more serious issue: the link between childhood obesity and chronic adult disease.

We now know that obesity is a definite risk factor for a number of diseases, including heart disease and stroke, high blood pressure, cancer, Type II diabetes, gallbladder disease, and for complications from any type of surgery. Recent studies from researchers highlight the enormity and the seriousness of the obesity epidemic:

- The Centers for Disease Control tells us that obesity is becoming a national health problem with nearly 15 percent—*almost nine million children*—now categorized as seriously overweight, and that number is rising. Instead of seeing heart disease occur when our children reach their fifties and sixties, researchers are predicting that our sons and daughters might be subject to heart disease as early as their twenties and thirties.

- A recent study published in the *New England Journal of Medicine* showed a direct relationship between excess weight and the risk of death from most cancers—the more body fat our children carry, the greater their risk.

- Researchers from Duke University report that a staggering number of obese children are developing Type II diabetes earlier in their lives, in some cases, during their teenage years.

What can we do about these findings? We need to prevent our children from becoming obese—that means ensuring that they eat nutritious foods and exercise regularly. If they have already started down the path to obesity we need to intervene immediately. If we can prevent a child from becoming an obese adult, we will be making a substantial difference in their lives.

Obesity is a vitally important issue, so let's be clear. Many confuse obesity with a few stubborn pounds—but it's not those extra five pounds everyone wants to lose. According to the National Institute of Health and the Centers for Disease Control and Prevention, individuals are considered obese when their weight is 20 percent or more over the maximum desirable for their height. Obesity is also defined as a BMI (body mass index) over 30. Adults with a BMI between 25 and 29.9 are considered overweight, but not obese. In children, obesity is also defined as a BMI equal to or greater than the 95th percentile on the BMI graph. (To learn how to calculate BMI, turn to The Tools, page 157.)

Stop Heart Disease in its Tracks

Our children may be overeating their way to heart disease. According to the American Heart Association, the increasing epidemic of obesity among children is setting them up for cardiovascular disease later in life. To prevent this from happening, they recommend that we do everything we can to stop our children from becoming obese as early as possible.

Do you know how a heart attack occurs? How about a stroke? Heart attacks occur when coronary arteries clog. Fat, traveling through the arteries, builds up and attaches to the coronary artery walls. The accumulation of fat creates fatty streaks, which change into plaque. Plaque creates clots in the artery that reduce the flow of blood to the heart. A stroke occurs when an artery that goes to the brain becomes clogged, or when a blood vessel in the brain ruptures.

We now know that too much dietary fat—particularly saturated fat and trans fats—and too much cholesterol, play a major role in the buildup of those thin, white fatty streaks that ultimately lead to heart attack and stroke. Since our children are now showing evidence of these fatty streaks as young as ten years old, it's essential that we cut down on fat.

Along with too much saturated fat, trans fat, and cholesterol, an iron excess may also prove to be a risk factor for heart disease, particularly for our sons. Our bodies can use only a normal amount of iron. Iron that isn't used is stored as excess. We are now associating such excess iron with an increased risk of heart disease. Unlike our sons, after puberty, the risk for our daughters diminishes: when they begin to menstruate the excess iron is discharged monthly in blood. This may be one reason why coronary artery disease is less common in women (pre-menopausal) than men.

High Blood Pressure/Hypertension— Bringing Down the Risk

To better understand how high blood pressure develops and leads to hypertension and heart disease you need look no further than salt and its effect on the body. Too much salt causes our kidneys to react. To excrete excess salt, the kidneys increase our body's blood pressure. Continued elevated blood pressure leads to hypertension, which is a major risk factor for coronary artery disease and stroke.

American children are showing increases in both weight and blood pressure levels. Right now, an estimated 10 to 15 percent of school-age children have high blood pressure for their age, and the numbers are rising. These percentages parallel the obesity epidemic and the increased consumption of salty snacks and fast foods in young children around the world.

Children aren't born with a taste for salt. That's right—it's actually an acquired taste. And the sad fact is that we Americans consume ten times as much salt as we need. It's in our frozen foods, our canned foods, our processed foods, our snack foods, and also on the dinner table. It's everywhere! So why not put those saltshakers away now and help our children avoid high blood pressure and a lifetime on expensive drugs with possible side effects?

Type II Diabetes—A Threat to *All* Our Children

Over the past twenty years, Type II diabetes has increased dramatically in both children and adults. That enormous increase has now been linked to childhood obesity. The lack of physical activity isn't helping either. Our kids are spending more than thirty-eight hours a week watching TV, playing video games, downloading music, or chatting with friends on computers—anything but exercising!

How does childhood obesity link to Type II diabetes? It's all about fat cells. Overweight children are not able to either produce or to utilize all the insulin they need to keep their bodies energized. Insulin must find its way inside all the cells of the body to do its work. Fat cells are the most difficult to penetrate, and an obese child has too many fat cells for insulin to work properly. To compensate, the pancreas begins to produce as much insulin as it can, but eventually the amount needed will remain inadequate and the symptoms of diabetes will appear.

In the past, this disease has typically shown up after the age of thirty. But the 2001 Obesity Statistics from the U.S. government tell us that one in four overweight children is already showing early signs of Type II diabetes, and that 60 percent of these children already have one risk factor for heart disease.

Although these new statistics are distressing, they also clarify what must be done to protect our children. We must help prevent our children from becoming obese! And if they're already obese, let's help them lose the excess fat and reverse the symptoms of Type II diabetes.

Cancer—A Deadly Disease With Childhood Roots

To all of us, cancer is perhaps the most frightening of diseases. If we thought that lessening our children's risk of developing cancer as adults was within our reach, which of us wouldn't do everything possible to make it happen? Well, we now know that by changing the foods we offer our children, we may be able to lower their risk potential for cancer.

There's no magic bullet, but we do have a fantastic opportunity to give our kids the best protection. The new research tells us that our best chance is an anticancer diet low in total fat, high in dietary fiber and in certain vitamins, all found in fruits and vegetables. In fact, if only one dietary change were to be initiated to reduce the risk of cancer, the best would be to eat a more colorful mix of fruits and vegetables like blueberries, pumpkin, mango, apricots, peaches, oranges, tomatoes, sweet potatoes, carrots, broccoli, spinach, dark leafy greens, and watercress. These foods are low in calories, low in fat (particularly saturated fat), free of cholesterol, high in fiber and in beta-carotene (a form of vitamin A), vitamin C, and natural cancer-fighting compounds.

Osteoporosis—Bank Enough Bone for a Lifetime

Is there any parent among us who doesn't want to stay physically fit and active throughout our lives? And is there any parent who doesn't long for that same mobility for their children as they age? Of course—no one wants their children to experience hip or vertebrae fractures in the future.

Childhood is a unique period for preventing osteoporosis. It is the ideal time for building and storing reserves of good bone. From pregnancy to early adult life, more bone is being formed than is being lost. Subsequently, from our early thirties for women and early forties for men, more bone is being lost than deposited.

We've all heard over and over again that calcium is the key to building strong bones. That's why it's imperative that we give our children the maximum amount of calcium to protect them from bone loss as they age and instill in them the importance of exercise in building strong bones. This is especially important for our daughters, who are ten times more likely to suffer osteoporosis later in life than our sons. After menopause, bone loss increases again. If we haven't deposited good bone reserves in childhood, our daughters won't have enough bone to draw on for support and will end up with thin, weak, brittle bones—the hallmark of osteoporosis.

I hope you now have a clearer picture and a deeper understanding of that critical link between the foods we feed our children and their risk of developing chronic adult diseases.

The challenge doesn't have to be complicated. It's up to all of us to become proactive parents and dedicate ourselves to lowering our children's risk for these diseases. By making the necessary nutritional and lifestyle changes, it can be done.

I strongly believe that whether you're expecting a child, are the parent of a newborn, a toddler, a school-age child, or an adolescent, if they're under your guidance, then you still have the chance to offer them the gift of a healthy, disease-free life.

This is a great place to start!

2

You *Can* Lower the Risk of Childhood Obesity

All of us soften and smile when we see a small child with well-padded arms, dimpled cheeks, and chubby little thighs. And that's the way babies are supposed to look, just like that adorable Gerber baby who's been smiling out at us from baby food jars for so many years.

Max and Kate were actually good-size babies for twins, weighing in at 6 pounds 11 ounces and 5 pounds 14 ounces, respectively. And by the age of 3 months, they had more than doubled in size! Max weighed 15 pounds 11 ounces, and Kate weighed 14 pounds 13 ounces at their three month doctor's appointment. Genuinely concerned, we asked the doctor, "Are they too big? Are we feeding them too much?" Our doctor smiled and said, "Babies this little really can't be overfed because when they're full they stop eating or spit up, unlike us." Too bad we all couldn't retain that sensibility as we grow up!

But, of course, as babies grow into the toddler years, there comes a time when some of us ask, "Will she outgrow that baby fat with age?" What we should really be asking, however, is, "Is she eating too much? Is she eating the right foods? Is she getting enough exercise? Will she grow into a healthy adult?"

These are valid concerns. While we've all been living fast-paced lives, turning to drive-thrus with super-size meals more and more often, obesity has caught up with

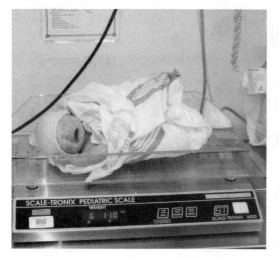 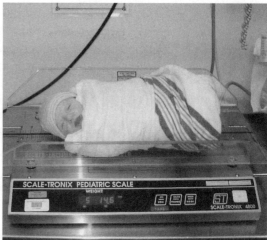

Max weighs in.   *Kate weighs in.*

many of our children. And it has now become a national epidemic. Obesity is so pervasive that many health professionals are referring to our children as Generation O. In fact, according to the head of the Centers for Disease Control and Prevention, obesity is the number one health threat in the United States today. Among children and teens, ages 6 to 19, almost nine million are overweight and over 10 percent of younger preschool children, ages 2 to 5, are also overweight. And these numbers are rising!

Compounding the problem, obesity is beginning to show itself earlier and earlier. More teens are now overweight than at any time in history: our children are now acquiring midlife paunches at the age of 10! And I don't have to tell you that the risk for school yard ridicule is a given—fat just isn't "cool." This social stigma can lower a child's self-esteem, and can leave them with lasting emotional scars.

But more importantly, as Dr. Winick points out, obesity presents our children with a risk for serious chronic adult diseases—heart disease and stroke, high blood pressure, Type II diabetes, and cancer. It's reason enough for all of us as parents to be rightfully concerned, if not downright worried.

How It Works: Fat is a tissue. In fact, it's one of the largest tissues in our body, normally making up from 5 to 20 percent of our total body tissue mass. As our children grow, they're continually adding more cells to every tissue in their bodies. Fat tissue itself is made up of millions of fat cells, each containing a small globule of fat in its center.

Obesity, or too much fat in the body, can occur in two different ways: each fat cell can be swollen with too large a fat globule (as happens when adults gain weight), or there can be too many fat cells (containing normal-size globules). Childhood obesity results in *too many* fat cells. It's very important for all parents to understand that *once a fat cell forms it will remain for life.* Weight loss will reduce the size of the fat globule, but it will never reduce the number of fat cells. That means that a child with too many fat cells will only be able to lose weight by reducing the amount of fat in each cell. Why is this significant? Since an obese child will never lose fat cells and can only decrease the size of the existing fat cells, she can only attain a healthy weight by reducing the amount of fat in the fat cells so that they are ultimately *below* the normal size. This type of weight loss is *very* difficult to maintain.

By contrast, with adult-onset obesity, the number of fat cells is normal. It is their size that's too large. When we adults lose weight, unlike our children, we reduce the size of our fat cells, leaving the fat tissue in a normal condition. So childhood obesity not only leads to adult obesity, but it also leads to a very difficult form of obesity to treat. Obviously, the best approach is to prevent this form of obesity from ever occurring.

Normal Non-Obese

Childhood Obesity
Too Many Fat Cells

Adult Obesity
Fat Cells Too Large

The Fat Dilemma

None of us wants to believe that our adorable child is obese. It's easier to assume that her excess fat will just melt away as she grows taller, but that may be wishful thinking. Dr. Winick tells us that an obese child over the age of four has an 80 percent chance of becoming an obese adult—and that statistic, like excess fat, is difficult to wish away.

Without intervention or treatment, most fat children are on their way to becoming fat adults. That is the unpleasant truth. Worse, it's much more difficult to treat an obese adult who was an obese child than to treat a person who became obese in their adult years.

The Genetics Connection

The genetics connection is loaded with surprises—it influences where fat is stored in the body, how quickly hunger is satisfied, and which of our children will have the greater chance of becoming obese. Understanding what puts our children at higher risk is an important piece to the whole obesity puzzle. If one parent is obese, a child has a 40 percent chance of becoming obese. If both parents are obese, the risk jumps to 80 percent.

Recently, a particular genetic defect in childhood obesity was partially identified—a subtle difference in the resting metabolic rate.

How It Works: To get a better picture of what the resting metabolic rate actually means, think of the body as a machine. The resting metabolic rate is the energy expended as the machine idles. When the body idles or is at rest, like the machine, it too is still expending energy: the energy necessary for the heart to beat, the lungs to breathe, the muscles to maintain their tone, and for the body's temperature to remain at 98.6 degrees Fahrenheit. Some of us expend less energy than others to maintain these vital functions. But no matter how many calories are taken in, the less energy we expend, the more calories are left over. What happens to those calories? They're stored as fat! That means that the person who expends the fewest calories to maintain the "running motor" may be more efficient metabolically, but is at greater risk for obesity. Yep, as unfair as it seems, those extra calories will be converted to fat.

So what does it mean to be metabolically efficient? Calories are burned at a much slower rate. In a society where food is scarce, the more metabolically efficient person needs fewer calories to survive than the less metabolically efficient person who burns calories at a faster rate. But food isn't scarce in our society, and eating excess calories is an everyday proposition. This is bad news for the person who burns calories slowly. Even though not all obese people overeat, they do overeat in comparison to what they need to burn, and it may be even less than what their much leaner friends consume. And it all goes back to that resting metabolic rate.

Successful prevention and treatment of childhood obesity depend on understanding and utilizing these facts.

The Home Connection

We all know that family members share the same genes, but they also share the same diets, ethnic food preferences, behavioral eating patterns, meal and snacking routines, and activities. Some families eat all their meals together around a table, others eat on the run, standing at the kitchen counter, or staring at the television. No matter how, when, or where the family eats, our children accept the pattern they see as normal and mimic that behavior. And it's not always to our children's advantage.

For example Gwen, a Long Island teacher, has been worried for some time about her ten-year-old son, Tim, who has been gradually gaining weight. While she and her husband are still at work, Tim returns from school, sits in front of his computer, and munches on potato chips, cookies, frozen pizza, ice cream—all the fast-food snacks the family loves to eat. Although Tim is aware he's growing larger and his weight is beginning to affect his self-esteem, he continues eating and playing computer games. A little investigation makes it clear that Tim is mirroring the eating and activity habits of his parents.

When Gwen and her husband, Harold, come home, they have a vodka and tonic and snack on corn chips and sour cream dip. Since everyone's tired, they might go out to McDonald's for burgers and fries, and when they return home, plunk themselves down in recliners and on the couch to watch TV. That's when Gwen pulls out the coffee cake and ice cream.

Tim isn't the only one Gwen should be worrying about. At five feet seven inches, she has ballooned to 192 pounds. Harold, who used to be a bantamweight boxer, weighing in at 150, has just tipped the scales at 215. A loving family, they laugh at their burgeoning waistlines, half-heartedly promising to start making some changes—tomorrow.

Our children learn by our example, not by our intentions. This would be a perfect time for Gwen, Harold—and Tim—to set conscious eating guidelines and to devise a healthy food plan for the family. Intervening on Tim's weight gain may shield him from many of the obesity-related diseases that could show up later in life.

The Exercise Connection

It's not just the additional calories our children are consuming that's making them obese. Many experts now believe that in addition to the food they eat—sodas, French fries, pizza, triple cheeseburgers, chips, doughnuts, high-fat ice cream, and cookies—the other major reason for the childhood obesity epidemic is a lack of exercise. Our children simply aren't running, jumping, and moving their bodies like kids used to before television and computers came along. It also hasn't helped that schools have cut back on physical education programs to save on their budgets. And this downtime starts early—we're plopping our little ones down in front of video monitors even as young babies. So by the time they reach five, six, or seven, children are already glued to their computers and exercise is just not part of their vocabulary.

Well, it makes perfect sense when you consider that so many of us adults are also plopped in front of our computers and television sets, and our kids are mirroring our behavior. But did you know that watching TV might be a strong predictor of obesity? According to University of Minnesota researchers, television and video watching among both boys and girls is linked to the increased consumption of sodas, junk food—and obesity. As parents, we have introduced our children to the culture of sitting and watching. And until we get our children's lives more active again, we're going to have a very tough time beating this epidemic. We talked to physical fitness expert and martial arts master Beth Ann Bielat about this problem. She believes that, as parents, we should lead by example.

Beth Ann Bielat

Having taken on the job of being a parent, you now owe it to your child to teach him how to be healthy through exercise and diet. And don't wait for schools to take on this responsibility—this is YOUR baby!

Extensive research has proven that there are tremendous beneficial effects to being healthy and fit. Benefits include skeletal health and higher bone mineral density (BMD), better levels of blood lipids, more normal blood pressure, less body fat, and more lean body mass (muscle). Emotional and mental well-being have also been connected to health and fitness.

So let's start at the very beginning.

■ *Pregnancy*: It's not time to start a new, vigorous exercise program, but you can begin with walking, swimming, yoga, tai chi, and other moderate exercise. Your baby is already hearing your message of *leading by example* and getting the health benefits through you.

■ *Newborns and Infants*: Until about the age of four, you will not have any problem getting your child to move and exercise; however, once again, you must lead by example. These years are meant for walks, hikes, learning how to swim, and playing—lots and lots of playing!

■ *Young Children*: Around the age of four or five, you job as an exercise adviser begins. The President's Council on Physical Fitness and Sports recommends that a child be moderately active every day for at least one hour. It doesn't have to be concurrent—it can include a ten-minute walk, playing for a while after school, and swimming for fifteen minutes. Sedentary days should be few and far between.

It's very important to let your child try different activities to find out what she *loves.* I've always believed that the best exercise is the one your child will do! Introduce them to individual and group sports; let them experiment with swimming, soccer, basketball, karate, skateboarding, hiking, and dance.

It's also important for your children to succeed and feel good about themselves. If your child is the last one picked for a kickball team, he may hide from exercise for the rest of his life. I'm partial to martial arts, dance, and other activities that promote all the components of fitness, including strength, endurance, cardiovascular heath, flexibility, great coordination, motor skills, and proper body alignment. Find great teachers, coaches, and motivators.

■ *Adolescence:* Typically, this is when a lot of physical activity comes to a screeching halt. Daily participation declines greatly in males, but even more in females. Unfortunately, the biological drive to be active wanes and other factors become more prevalent, such as peer acceptance, physical capabilities, sexual attractiveness, and body image.

It can get even worse in college, where our children are newly independent, eating junk food, burdened with lots of homework, and spending too much time on the computer. Unless they have some healthy guidelines for eating and exercising, the extra pounds can just pour on. (I've seen many of my children's friends put on the "freshman fifteen!")

The more physically fit your children are at any age, the healthier they are at *all* ages. By getting your kids up and moving each and every day, you'll be giving them one of the greatest gifts in life—physical fitness, which will help to ensure quality of life and longevity.

Tracking Your Child's Risk for Obesity

How does a parent, any parent, find out if his child is at risk for childhood obesity? First, if either parent is obese, your child is at risk. And if both parents are obese, your child is at a higher risk. Second, if your child's rate of weight gain exceeds the rate of his increase in height, your child is at risk. To estimate the risk properly, your child's growth pattern must be monitored continually throughout childhood, not just during infancy.

Numerous graphs exist to plot the normal increase in height and weight for almost all children. During the first two years, these graphs are divided at monthly intervals, after that, at yearly intervals. Another graph shows the ratio of weight to height at any age. These graphs are included in "Part III—The Tools," so you can plot the progress of your children's growth.

HEIGHT AND WEIGHT CHARTS To determine whether your child is overweight, weight and height must be considered together. For example, let's say that your two-year-old son, Johnny, is growing in the fortieth percentile for his height and the fortieth percentile for his weight. That's just fine. If in a year, however, when Johnny is measured again, he's in the fortieth percentile for height but now in the fiftieth percentile for weight, that's a danger signal. And if his weight jumps to the sixtieth percentile, he's at high risk for obesity. Johnny may not yet fall into the obese category, but it's time to intervene. Now you can begin to see why it's so important to track your child's physical development.

It actually doesn't matter which percentile your child falls into (the sixtieth percentile means that forty percent of all children are taller or heavier, and sixty percent are shorter or lighter). Some children will be growing in the ninetieth percentile, while others will be growing in the tenth percentile. This is perfectly normal, since some children are tall and others are shorter; some are heavy while others are lighter. What you're looking for is for the percentile for both height and weight to remain constant.

To be absolutely clear, as soon as weight starts accelerating faster than height, your child could be moving toward obesity. And if your child falls into the ninety-fifth percentile in weight, he may need help.

STAGES OF GROWTH There are three distinct phases of growth in children: Infancy, middle childhood, and adolescence. (These phases are discussed in detail in Part II.) Because your child's diet is different during these periods, and because the stage of development is different, your methods of intervening to try to prevent childhood obesity should also be different. However, one general principle holds for infants, toddlers, and very young children. Your goal is not to get your young child to lose weight. Since younger children are growing and becoming taller, you really don't want to reduce their weight to prevent childhood obesity. Merely holding weight constant or allowing it to increase at a slower rate should accomplish the goal. However, older children who are overweight, especially those with a family history of obesity or other risk factors, should be considered for safe and appropriate dietary changes. Speak to your pediatrician.

THE BMI If you notice a change in percentiles—when weight is increasing significantly faster than height—it's a good time to ask your pediatrician to check your child's body mass index, otherwise called BMI.

BMI graphs use weight and height to estimate body fat and gauge health risks associated with carrying too much weight. These graphs are not regularly used for children, though; only for those whose weight is increasing significantly faster than height. To routinely plot your child's growth for her first two years, you'll want to use the standard tables that show height and weight for age. After two years, you'll use height and weight tables for ages 2–20. However, if your child's weight is increasing faster than height between ages 2 and 3, you'll want to get a baseline BMI percentile for your child from your pediatrician, a percentile against which all future ratios will be compared. Again, this isn't a routine measurement—most pediatricians only use the BMI on children who are too fat or too thin because it's a more accurate diagnostic tool.

To help you plot your child's growth, you'll find all the necessary charts and instructions in "Part III—The Tools."

It's Never Too Early to Lower the Risk of Childhood Obesity

We know now that the causes of childhood obesity are complex, that there is cause for concern, and that the solution is not something that will occur overnight. But by making changes now, staying conscious of our family's food dynamics and exercise activities, and by carefully tracking our children's changes in growth patterns, we will be giving our kids a greater chance to live longer, healthier lives.

3

You *Can* Protect Your Child from the Risk of Heart Disease

Are you one of those parents who believe that heart disease doesn't begin developing until middle age? If you answered yes, you're not alone. When the words *heart attack, stroke,* or *atherosclerosis* are mentioned, most of us think of people in their sixties or older. However, we now know that the signs of heart disease actually begin developing during childhood, and that we have it in our power to lower our children's risk and possibly even prevent them from becoming heart-sick adults. That's why it's vital to understand the importance of gathering a family medical history and also to realize the dangerous role that fat-laden diets play in the development of plaque in our children's arteries. (Other major risk factors include obesity, Type II diabetes, hypertension, and smoking, and are discussed in detail in other chapters.)

One morning on *GMA,* we had a doctor from the American Heart Association on the show who went through a checklist for viewers to use to find out if they were at risk for heart disease. As he went through the checklist, my blood pressure started rising: I wasn't faring so well. I wasn't as active as I should be. I weighed more than I knew I should weigh. And I thought that there had been some relatives in my family who had had heart disease—but I really wasn't sure because I hadn't gathered my family medical information properly. Adding it all up became a major turning point in my life. It was as if the checklist had grabbed me by my collar, shook me, and said: "You *must* take responsibility here. You *must* understand that you flunked this test. You *must* be able to retake this test in a year or two and pass it! Because if you don't, you're not going to have a healthy life, and you're not going to be around to play with your kids." That's when I started paying attention to my diet, adding exercise into my routine, and asking my mom questions about our family.

Today, with this new research in hand, it has become more evident than ever that what we inherit from our family and the eating patterns that we develop as we grow up will determine whether we fall prey to heart disease.

Dr. W | Tracking Fatty Streaks

The most frequent type of heart disease is hardening of the arteries, or atherosclerosis. As I mentioned in my Passionate Plea to Parents, during the Korean and Vietnam wars, when autopsies were performed on soldiers who died in battle, the doctors were surprised to find fatty streaks in the coronary arteries of more than half of the young American soldiers, but not in the Korean or Vietnamese soldiers. Back then, heart disease was felt to be the domain of the elderly, so doctors were surprised to see fatty streaks—the earliest signs of coronary heart disease—show up in men in their early twenties. Sadly, we're now seeing heart disease starting even earlier. In numerous studies, fatty streaks have been found in the arteries of young teenaged boys in an alarmingly high number. Even more frightening are the findings of a lengthy study of sixteen thousand children, conducted in Bogalusa, Louisiana, between 1972 and 1997. Researchers in the Bogalusa Heart Study found evidence of fatty streaks in children as young as five years old!

Heart Disease Begins in Childhood

It would be wonderful if we had X-ray vision and could see into the workings of our children's hearts. We'd be able to see that some of our sons and daughters are developing fatty streaks in their arteries at ten years of age, and sometimes even earlier. Although we can't visually track our children's arteries, we can make some critical nutritional changes.

How It Works: It all starts with a little fatty streak, a small deposit of fat inside the inner lining of a coronary artery where the blood flows to the heart. Cholesterol (fat) builds up in the narrow artery tubes, creating a substance called plaque. Over time, the plaque accumulates more fat deposits, narrowing the inside opening of the artery even more, and eventually a blood clot may form that blocks off blood flow to the heart. If the heart is deprived of blood and oxygen, a heart attack may occur.

A stroke begins with the same fatty streaks, but instead of blocking the arteries to the heart, they block the arteries to the brain.

The Good and the Bad Cholesterol

Those cholesterol (fat) deposits in the arteries cause blockages of blood to the heart, but what exactly is cholesterol, and what's the difference between the good and bad cholesterol we've heard so much about?

Cholesterol is a waxy, fat-like substance naturally produced by the liver. Our bodies need cholesterol to help with the production of hormones and vitamin D, and to assist with the building of cell walls. Our bodies naturally produce all of the cholesterol we need. But we also consume cholesterol, which comes from meat and poultry, dairy products and eggs.

How It Works: Much like trying to mix oil and water, cholesterol (oil) and blood, a watery-based material, just won't mix. Cholesterol (and other lipids) will not dissolve in blood. Instead, the cholesterol circulates, attached to a much larger group of molecules called lipoproteins, which serve as the boats that carry the cholesterol in the plasma. The lipoprotein navy consists mainly of two kinds of vessels that are described by their density: low-density lipoprotein (LDL) and high-density lipoprotein (HDL). Seventy percent of the navy is LDL and 30 percent is HDL. These two ships have different functions. LDL carries cholesterol to the tissues and may spill cholesterol into atherosclerotic plaques. HDL carries cholesterol from the cells and, it is believed, out of the arterial plaques. Every cell in the body contains docks for LDL, known as receptors.

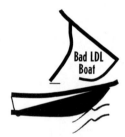

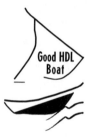

Carrying Fat Into the Arteries   *Taking Fat Out of the Arteries*

As you'll see, children have lower levels of cholesterol, particularly the bad LDL, than adults. This Serum Cholesterol chart shows the differences between children in their midyears and adults. (Serum is the clear fluid part of blood in which cholesterol moves through the body.)

Serum Cholesterol Levels

	Desirable	Borderline	High
Child	Below 170	170–199	Anything Above 200
Adult	Below 200	200–239	Anything Above 240

Homocysteine Levels—A New Risk Factor

Another cause of heart disease, recently discovered, is high levels of a circulating amino acid called homocysteine. These high levels are usually due to inadequate dietary intake of the vitamin folic acid. However, poor dietary intake of vitamins B_{12} or B_6 may also result in high homocysteine levels.

Our concern about elevated homocysteine levels is new and important. By giving our children adequate folic acid, we may be able to avoid yet another possible risk factor for heart disease. It may be as simple as adding dark leafy greens (like kale and spinach), asparagus, dried beans, oranges, and orange juice, and whole grains to our children's meals.

The Genetic Connection

If there is a family history of early heart disease (age forty or fifty), your child is at risk for developing it. In families where one or both parents have a history of high cholesterol levels (hypercholesterolemia), readings above 200, or an LDL level above 160, your child is at risk for developing high cholesterol. The higher the level of LDL cholesterol, the greater your child's risk. Have your child tested if your family has such a history—the earlier the better. Dr. Winick advises, however, that most children don't need to be screened, especially if you adopt a diet low in fat and cholesterol after your child is four years of age.

The Iron Connection

Although cholesterol seems to be the major culprit in our children's risk for heart disease, a few other nutrients may also be involved. Since the early 1980s, scientists have questioned the relationship between high levels of stored iron and heart disease. While the relationship is still being investigated, a recent Finnish study indicates that excess iron may be a risk factor for coronary artery disease especially in males.

Iron is required for normal growth and development, which means that iron requirements for both boys and girls are particularly high. Because iron is an integral part of the hemoglobin in the red blood cell, a deficiency in iron will lead to a deficiency of hemoglobin, which is anemia.

No one wants her child to be anemic. Anemia can lead to irritability, restlessness, poor attention span, tiredness, poor athletic performance, and in severe cases, shortness of breath. To avoid these symptoms, we often give our children vitamins containing iron, and fortified breakfast cereals. But this may be too much. The body hoards iron very well, and excess iron reserves could lead our sons to early heart disease. By contrast, the risk to our daughters is less; once menstruation begins, they deplete their iron stores. Since heart disease is a leading killer in more men than women, these findings have caused pediatricians to reevaluate the entire subject of iron supplementation. Boys and girls must be supplemented differently. As parents, we want to prevent iron deficiencies, but before we supplement our older children with iron, let's check out their risk factors with our pediatricians. On the bright side, most of our children will not become iron deficient if we feed them a healthy, balanced diet.

It's Never Too Early to Protect Your Child from the Risk of Heart Disease

Since cardiovascular disease is at near epidemic proportions in the United States, we need to take this information to heart. As parents, let's start by decreasing the amount of saturated fats and trans fats in our children's diets, and simultaneously begin increasing the amounts of whole grains, fruits, vegetables, fish, and the degree of physical activity. This is a great way for the entire family to become heart healthy.

4

You *Can* Minimize Your Child's Risk of High Blood Pressure

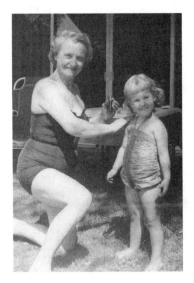

Me at four with my grandma Lila, who had high blood pressure.

When you were growing up and eating meals with your family, was the saltshaker always on the table? Did anyone in your family add salt to food without even tasting it first? Did anyone automatically add a little more salt after tasting the food whether it needed it or not? I can tell you, my grandmother did! She also had high blood pressure, hypertension, and ultimately died of heart disease. My mother also was pretty good friends with her saltshaker. As for me, about ten years ago when I became educated about salt, I stopped cooking with it and I stopped putting the saltshaker on the dinner table. Nonetheless, my daughters have continued to ask for that saltshaker. It's a constant debate, one in which I'm always asking for a salt treaty!

How does this preference for salt come about? Is it inborn or is it learned? And what effect does all this salt have on our bodies?

High Blood Pressure Begins in Childhood

Does hypertension have its roots in childhood? The simple answer to this question is yes! There are two conditions that lead to hypertension. The first is obesity, which, as we've seen, can have its roots in childhood. And the second is consuming too much sodium, which is present in its greatest quantity as salt (sodium chloride). A pretty conclusive body of evidence exists that tells us that the consumption of large amounts of salt (in both animal and human populations) can result in elevated blood pressure.

- There is abundant evidence demonstrating that obese children, as well as obese adults, have higher systolic and diastolic blood pressure when compared to children and adults of normal weight.

- Animal studies show that certain strains of rats with normal blood pressure develop hypertension shortly after salt is added to their diet.

- In countries where low-salt diets are the norm, blood pressure is lower and does not increase as the population ages. In countries where high-salt diets are the norm (United States, Japan, and Western Europe), blood pressure is higher and increases with age.

- When men on low-salt diets from certain African countries were drafted into the army and were introduced to high-salt meals, they rapidly developed hypertension. Even after they had completed their military duty and resumed their low-salt diets (*not* no-salt), the hypertension persisted.

- Before antihypertension drugs were used, a famous program at Duke University treated people with high blood pressure with a no-salt, low-sodium food diet. Most of the participants significantly lowered their blood pressure.

- During a study on newborns and infants, a tiny bit of salt was placed on their tongues. They would spit it out, grimace, and often cry. When the same was done with sugar, these infants smiled and swallowed.

Since newborn infants will reject salty foods, when and how does this preference for salty food develop? It develops as a result of constant exposure to salty foods, and it can begin in early infancy.

As parents, we should be very aware that too much salt intake and obesity are the culprits behind the new epidemic of high blood pressure that we're seeing in our children.

- A recent study conducted in the Netherlands found that children who had been on low-salt diets during the first six months of their lives had lower blood pressures than those children who had been on normal sodium diets. When these same children were checked again after fifteen years, the low-salt group still had lower blood pressures.

- The American Heart Association reports that the growing rate of obesity may be contributing to the unexpected increase in the number of children with high blood pressure.

How It Works: Blood circulates through the arteries of the body as a result of the pumping action of the heart. Since the heart alternately contracts and relaxes, two levels of blood pressure can be recorded. So when we measure our blood pressure, we are measuring the pressure of the blood flow inside the arteries.

The top number (systolic) records the pressure exerted against the arteries during the contraction phase of the heartbeat. The bottom number (diastolic) records the pressure exerted between contractions, when the heart muscle is relaxed. An elevation in either reading—the top or bottom numbers—tells us that more strain is being placed on the arteries than normal. This strain is called high blood pressure. An elevated pressure, especially an elevated diastolic number, can lead to damaged arteries and organs. Persistent high blood pressure (called hypertension) is dangerous in that it increases our risk of heart attack and stroke.

A typical blood pressure reading for a healthy adult would be 120/80. The systolic or contracting number is 120; the diastolic or relaxing number is 80.

In children, both the systolic and diastolic pressures are lower. The younger the child, the lower the pressure. When the blood pressure is too low, not enough blood reaches the tissues. The brain, which is most sensitive to this reduction in blood supply, reacts by causing dizziness, and even loss of consciousness. By contrast, when the blood pressure is too high, there may be no symptoms, but the large and small arteries can be damaged by constant exposure to these higher than normal pressures.

Two types of responses may result, both very dangerous. First, an artery may rupture. If a rupture occurs in an artery feeding the brain, the person suffers one type of stroke, a cerebral hemorrhage. If the arterial wall becomes damaged, it becomes easier for lipids (fat) to be deposited, and atherosclerosis can occur. The artery eventually becomes blocked (or "occluded"), and blood flow is diminished to certain vital organs. If this occurs in the brain, the brain tissue normally fed by the blocked artery dies, and another type of stroke occurs. If an artery feeding part of the heart is blocked, we refer to this as a heart attack. Depending on the size of the artery and the portion of the heart it supplies, the person may die, or may recover with a damaged heart, or may recover with only minor heart damage. So the danger of hypertension is that it increases the risk of heart attack and stroke.

The Genetic Connection—and Other Risk Factors

When determining your child's risk for high blood pressure as an adult, Dr. Winick tells us that genetics must be taken into consideration. If there is a history of high blood pressure in your family, particularly in the histories of parents or grandparents, your child must be considered at risk. So take the time to complete the Family Health Tree and Work Sheet in Part III, "The Tools." You'll be glad you did.

Another genetic factor is race: African-American children of both sexes are at higher risk than Caucasian or Asian children. Also, a child born with a low birth weight is at increased risk as well. And yet again, *childhood obesity is a major risk factor!*

If your child falls into any of these groups, or if your child's blood pressure tends to be high, ask your doctor to monitor the pressure, especially if more than a year has passed since the last checkup. All children should have their blood pressure measured at their regular checkups. Request the actual numbers, systolic and diastolic, the top and bottom numbers.

Normal Blood Pressure Chart

Age Boys and Girls	Systolic Pressure MM Hg (Top Number)	Diastolic Pressure MM Hg (Bottom Number)
6 to 9 years	< 111	< 70
10 to 12 years	< 117	< 75
13 to 15 years	< 124	< 77
Adults	< 130	< 85

Key: < less than

Hypertension Chart *High - Significant - Severe*

Age	High Normal MM Hg	Significant Hypertension MM Hg	Severe Hypertension MM Hg
6 to 9 years			
Systolic (upper)	111–121	122–129	> 129
Diastolic (lower)	70–77	70–85	> 85
10 to 12 years			
Systolic (upper)	117–125	126–133	> 133
Diastolic (lower)	75–81	82–89	> 89
13 to 15 years			
Systolic (upper)	124–135	136–143	> 143
Diastolic (lower)	75–81	86–91	> 91
16 to 18 years			
Systolic (upper)	Not Given	140–179	> 179
Diastolic (lower)	Not Given	90–109	> 109

Key: > greater than

If your child's pressure constantly hovers around the higher levels of normal, he might have an increased risk for developing hypertension later in life. It's a good idea to keep a record of these blood pressure numbers.

The Salt Impact

Once again, when consumed in excess, calories and sodium will increase a child's risk for developing hypertension later in life. We've talked a lot about consuming too many calories, but in our society, we also consume ten times as much salt as we need. And we don't need that much. If we restricted our sodium intake to what is naturally found in foods, we would still have enough. The best rule of thumb is to consume foods as they are and not to add too much salt—no more than a teaspoon in a twenty-four-hour period. This includes salt from all foods, including chips, pretzels, popcorn, and prepared foods.

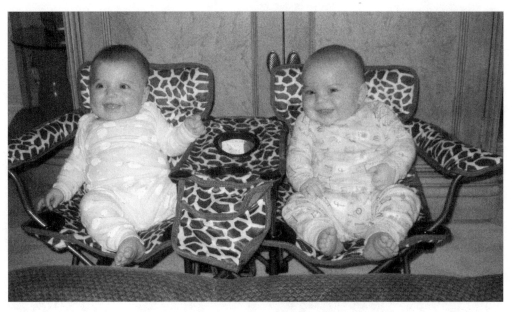

Kate and Max, already a happy team. And wiser than we know!

THE WISDOM OF BABIES Years ago the baby food industry added salt to many of their foods. Why? They knew infants didn't like salt. They even knew that adding salt was not in the best interest of most infants. But they also knew that mothers quite often tasted the food before giving it to their children. Since unsalted food tasted bland, and since the taste of salt was preferred, mothers would buy the product that was salted. It was only when mothers began to understand that added salt might be harmful that consumer opinion changed. Subsequently, consumers pressured the industry, and this resulted in baby foods finally being prepared without the salt.

Babies have a wisdom adults have forgotten. They instinctively know that salt will overwhelm their little bodies. Yes, there was a time when the iodine in salt was an important part of our diet. In the early 1920s, salt was first fortified with iodine to prevent goiters—overgrown thyroid glands. Today, we don't need to salt our foods for the iodine benefit. We consume sufficient amounts of iodine in tuna, canned and fresh fish, cheese, and processed foods.

So what part does salt play in the development of high blood pressure?

How It Works: High blood pressure is intimately linked to salt intake and the healthy functioning of our kidneys. As the blood circulates throughout the kidneys, many substances, including sodium, which we get almost entirely from salt, are filtered out. When too much sodium is present, the filtering process is unable to handle the heavy load without blood pressure increasing.

When the kidneys become tired and overworked and high blood pressure is persistent, simply eliminating salt won't solve the problem. At that point, prescribed medication may be required for life. It's much easier to prevent high blood pressure than to control it.

Remember, babies don't like salt, babies don't need added salt, and babies can live perfectly well without it. Thankfully, today's commercial baby foods cater to infants and not their parents, and so are made without additional salt. If you're making your own baby food at home, be careful when blending table foods. Ask yourself: are these foods salted to reflect my family's preferences? If your answer is yes, keep in mind that those foods are helping your child to develop a preference for salt, and with it, an increased risk for high blood pressure.

As our children get older, they'll be bombarded with highly salty foods— hamburgers, French fries, pizza, potato chips, pretzels, and a long list of other so-called fun foods. And, of course, children watch their parents. If Dad adds salt before eating, your child figures it must be right and will add salt also. That means that by example we're teaching them a lesson that's setting them up for high blood pressure, hypertension, heart attack, and stroke.

Certain foods loaded with salt should be limited, such as anything pickled, cured, or smoked. Get in the habit of reading labels, making use of salt substitutes, and cooking with other seasonings and flavors that will add taste but not sodium. Finally, beware of hidden sources of sodium such as those in frozen foods, prepared foods, canned foods, and salty snack foods.

It's Never Too Early to Minimize Your Child's Risk of High Blood Pressure

We can help prevent our children from developing high blood pressure by refusing to introduce our infants to salt, and by offering our older children tasty alternatives. We can also help them (and ourselves) by using less salt in the meals we prepare, by taking the saltshaker off the table, and by not cultivating their taste for salty foods.

5

You *Can* Diminish Your Child's Risk of Developing Type II Diabetes

Type II diabetes has often been called the silent epidemic—with good reason. All too often we don't realize that it has developed until well after symptoms begin to occur. But now we're in a much better position to identify this disease in its earliest stages. And health care professionals all over the country are warning us: the rise in Type II diabetes in children is definitively linked to the growing epidemic of childhood obesity!

Today we know that family history and obesity are the two major components that will set children up for this disease. For me, family history played a big role in my awareness since I grew up watching this insidious disease ravage aunts on both sides of my family. They suffered from diabetes and died from its complications. As a result, I've been conscious of the risk factors for most of my life. I also informed my children's pediatri-

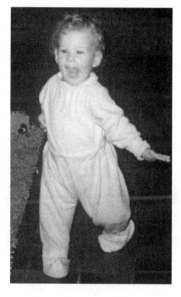

When I took my first steps and my first solids, the risks of Type II diabetes weren't as well known.

cian of our family history, and I'm especially careful about the foods we eat and the weight we gain. I know I can't do anything about my family history, but I can be diligent about protecting my children from the ravages of obesity and Type II diabetes. It's within our power to help our children prevent and reverse Type II diabetes, and it's up to us as parents to make sure that they eat right and exercise.

Many of you already know that Type II diabetes is also known as adult-onset diabetes. But according to researchers, that name is fast becoming an anachronism. The reason is glaring: more and more of our children are becoming overweight, and more and more of our children are getting this disease. Studies show that our sons and daughters are coming down with Type II diabetes eight to ten times more often than they did ten years ago.

Dr. W

When five-year-old Marc started kindergarten, he was in the eighty-fifth percentile for weight and height. By the fourth month of school, his parents began to notice that he was gaining a lot of weight but reasoned that he would just grow out of it. By the fifth month, Marc's teacher called his mother. "Marc is falling asleep during play and music," she said. "And he seems to be very hungry—when we have snacks, he always asks for seconds."

Marc's mother had been noticing that while at home, Marc showed no interest in playing outside with friends, and that he was continually plopped in front of the TV, napping and snacking. She had also noticed that he was drinking a great deal of liquids and going to the bathroom to urinate very often.

Concerned, she took Marc to see his pediatrician, who told her that Marc did indeed have a problem—he was in the early stages of Type II diabetes.

Obesity—a Major Key to Type II Diabetes

The message couldn't be clearer: when Type II diabetes is seen in children, it is almost exclusively in children who are obese. Along with the many other health risks that childhood obesity presents, a recent study from Yale University tells us that children with a significant degree of obesity are at a very high risk of developing Type II diabetes. Many obese children, some barely into preschool, are already starting to show the first signs of Type II diabetes.

Researchers at the University of North Carolina at Chapel Hill studied healthy, normal kids in five different schools. They determined which of the children showed one or more risk factors for Type II diabetes and then compared that information with their weight. Again, the only significant predictor they found was childhood obesity. Those children who were obese were fifty-three times as likely to have insulin resistance as those who were not obese.

So, make no mistake about it—as parents, obesity is our biggest concern. That's right, it's bigger than beer drinking, ear piercing, or tattoos. But along with this warning, let me give you the good news. The overwhelming number of children who lose the excess weight and are no longer considered obese, will also no longer be at risk for Type II diabetes.

Dr. W | **Type II Diabetes and the Special Dangers for Children**

In adults, Type II diabetes is always considered a serious disease. It not only increases the risk for heart attack and stroke, it also comes with its own set of complications. Since symptoms usually take years to develop, adults who get Type II diabetes in their sixties or seventies may never develop these complications. But it's a very different story for a child who develops Type II diabetes at age 15, or 10, or even younger, simply because she is obese. Unless that child's obesity is controlled, she has a whole lifetime to develop these complications. Not great news; however, the one ray of hope bears repeating: if your child's obesity is controlled and remains under control, then the diabetes almost always disappears. We don't know yet whether it will return much later in life (especially in those who are genetically prone), but think of the years you'll be adding to your child's life.

If your child is obese and develops Type II diabetes, treating the two conditions can become a difficult proposition. Both obesity and diabetes require some rather serious alterations in the diet—some changes are the same, but some are different. In essence, the child who is obese and has Type II diabetes will be on a much more restrictive diet than the obese child who doesn't have diabetes.

How It Works: Diabetes is a serious disease that's caused by either a deficiency in the amount of insulin or by the body's inability to utilize it. Insulin is an important hormone secreted by certain cells in the pancreas. It is needed by the body for, among other things, the conversion of certain nutrients—particularly the conversion of carbohydrates or fat into energy.

There are two types of diabetes. Type I, or juvenile diabetes, doesn't concern us here because nutrition plays no role in its cause. It occurs in certain genetically prone children who produce no insulin and must have daily insulin injections throughout their lives.

Type II diabetes, unlike Type I, is not a disease of the pancreas. Enough insulin is produced—in fact, sometimes more insulin is produced than in healthy people. The problem is different. The tissues of the body develop a resistance—a kind of auto-immunity—to the action of insulin. As a result, the amount of insulin produced is inadequate for the needs of the body. And there is a nutritional component to the development of this type of diabetes.

Insulin is very important to all the cells of the body. To convert carbohydrates and fat into energy, it must get inside the cells. Some cells are more easily penetrated than others. Fat cells are the most difficult to penetrate. Insulin receptors in fat cells are not as numerous and not as good at pulling the insulin in as other receptors. That means that the more fat cells our children have, the more insulin they need. That extra need for insulin causes the pancreas to produce more and more. But even with the pancreas producing all the insulin it can, the amount becomes inadequate. The cells sense this flood of insulin and become even more resistant. While the cells are starving for energy, the excess glucose accumulates and the symptoms of diabetes appear.

The Genetic Connection

The genetic component to Type II diabetes is very significant. If anyone in your immediate family—you or your spouse, grandparents, even an aunt or uncle—has diabetes, then your child is at risk.

In some cultures, the genetic connection is so high that just being a member of that culture increases the risk. For example, in several tribes of Native Americans, more than half the population either has or will develop diabetes, which, epidemiologically speaking, is astounding! Eastern-European Jews and African-Americans also have a genetic tendency to get adult-onset diabetes, however, the statistics are far less dramatic.

Dr. Winick points out, however, that if your family has a strong history of Type II diabetes, but your child's weight is normal, then there is no reason for testing. On the other hand, if your child is struggling with obesity, he or she must be tested even if there is no family history. In fact, *all obese children should be tested.* The test that your child should have is a fasting blood glucose level, and if this simple blood test shows a high glucose level, then more extensive blood tests (like a glucose tolerance test) should be done. Children who have the greatest chance of developing Type II diabetes are those who have a genetic predisposition to Type II diabetes—and are also obese.

The Sugar Problem

A child with Type II diabetes will need to be very careful about how much sugar she consumes. Although there is no evidence demonstrating that the quantity of sugar consumed leads to diabetes, feeding our children too many empty sugar calories can lead to obesity, a major risk factor for Type II diabetes, and a real danger for developing teeth.

It's Never Too Early to Diminish Your Child's Risk of Developing Type II Diabetes

The bottom line for us as parents is to understand that Type II diabetes in our children is directly associated with obesity. Since consuming excess calories is the only known nutritional factor causing the current epidemic, we'd better take this warning to alter our children's health to heart. And, of course, our children won't be the only ones to benefit from making healthy nutritional changes—reducing fat and calories will have a positive effect on the entire family.

Diabetes has a strong genetic connection for my family. That's why I took advantage of the Family Health Tree and Work Sheet, and I recommend that every parent do the same. I plan on giving each of my children a copy.

6

You *Can* Lessen Your Child's Risk of Cancer

Most children are blissfully unaware of cancer and cancer prevention, but the decisions that we, as parents, make about the foods they eat could determine whether they will stay blissfully unaffected or whether cancer will become a part of their future. The latest findings suggest that *nutritional factors are crucially important in causing almost all of the most common forms of cancer.* For all of us, this should be a loud wake-up call!

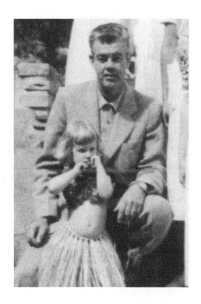

Me at two with my dad, who was a cancer surgeon.

My dad was a cancer surgeon, and when I was a little girl he used to take me to the hospital to make rounds with him and visit his patients. I remember he helped me with my first science project in school when I used plastic "Charlie Brown" figures to show the seven signs of cancer! My father devoted his life to finding a cure for cancer, but lamented that he didn't know if I'd see it in my lifetime. To me, what we're learning in this book is part of what my dad and other researchers have worked so hard to uncover: evidence that clearly links the foods we eat, the environment we live in, and the stresses to which we subject ourselves, to our increased chances of developing cancer. Sadly, my dad didn't live long enough to see this valuable information come to the forefront. When I was 13, he died in a plane crash returning from a national cancer conference. How gratified he would have been to have known that we now understand the link between nutrition and cancer, that things have begun to change in my lifetime . . . and that I'm involved in this exciting project to spread the news. What better legacy?

Dr. W | "Cancer Doesn't Just Suddenly Appear"

Cancer grows slowly. And this dreaded disease doesn't develop simply because of a lack of one single nutrient or an excess of another. We also know that it doesn't just suddenly appear. Cancer develops over time from dietary effects resulting from different nutrient combinations. Unlike focusing on fat as the obvious culprit behind heart disease, or on salt in the case of hypertension, to lessen the risk of cancer, we need to be focusing on the overall diets we feed our children.

The more we discover about the relationship between food and disease, the more we reshape the way we all think about cancer. Astounding new research tells us that 30 to 35 percent of all cancers can be attributed in part to diet. For example, eating fruits and vegetables has been linked to a decreased risk of lung, prostrate, bladder, esophagus, colorectal, and stomach cancers. Abundant evidence also tells us that excessive intake of fat from all sources will increase the incidence of cancer of the breast and colon. Many studies have shown that calorie excess and obesity are associated with most cancers, particularly cancer of the uterus and breast. Dietary fiber has been shown to protect against colon cancer and vitamin A (beta-carotene) against bladder cancer. Vitamins E and C have also been shown to reduce the risk for a number of cancers.

What kind of diet should we be feeding our children for maximum protection against cancer? A diet low in calories, low in fat, high in dietary fiber, high in vitamins A, E, and C— a diet with generous quantities of fruits and vegetables and other plant foods such as whole grains, beans, nuts, and seeds.

Our Growing Children and Cancer

Children are not small adults. Their growing organs increase in size by acquiring new cells—a process called cell division. In childhood, since all of the organs undergo continuous cell division, our children are more sensitive to the action of cancer-producing substances, especially those related to diet. What that means for us, as parents, is that childhood is the most important time—and the easiest—to influence our children's lifelong eating patterns.

How It Works Cancer isn't one disease. It's a group of diseases characterized by uncontrolled growth and spread of abnormal, or rebel, cells. A fundamental characteristic of cells is their ability to reproduce themselves by dividing. One cell becomes two, the two become four, and so on. The division of normal and healthy cells occurs systematically, replacing worn-out or injured cells. Conversely, cancer cells divide haphazardly and typically pile up into a nonstructured mass, or tumor, and compete with other bodily cells for nutrients.

The Genetic Connection

Many people believe that they've inherited the genetic potential for cancer and fear the worst. In fact, everyone has the genetic potential for the malignant transformation of any cell in their body—colon, lung, brain—all of them. However, malignant transformations usually don't occur by themselves but are typically the result of exposure to carcinogens through environment and diet. Only certain cancers are genetically predisposed—breast cancer has been shown to be one of them, especially if you are a tall and obese woman.

Unfortunately, there is no way to definitively assess your child's risk for cancer in later years. However, if you do have a history of cancer in your immediate family, adopting a diet low in fat with abundant fruits, and vegetables, and whole grains as early as possible is the best defense. And, of course, be sure to advise your pediatrician of your family history.

The Nutrition Connection

How does a poor diet work in the development of cancer? A poor diet probably stimulates cells with genes that have already been altered to grow into a tumor. In other words, a poor diet may not initiate cancer, but it can promote it.

How It Works Imagine a normal cell that's been damaged early in life from a genetic injury or from exposure to a cancer-causing chemical. When this damaged cell divides to form new cells, it passes along its damaged genetic material to those new cells. Remember, cancer doesn't just appear overnight—a tumor forms very slowly. But over time, a diet high in fat could promote the right kind of environment for a tumor to thrive.

Before long, what was once a single cell could become a tumor mass. That means that we may not be able to do much about the original damaged cell, but we may be able to decrease the tumor-promoting activity—*through diet*!

It's Never Too Early to Lessen Your Child's Risk of Cancer

Childhood is a critical time for establishing a cancer-preventing diet. This is the time in our children's lives when lifelong eating patterns are initiated, patterns that become difficult to break later on. Nowhere are dietary changes more important than in cancer prevention. Simply put, nutrition can help to build a sound defense that can help prevent cancer.

The recommended diet is not drastically different from the way most of us already eat, but it does require serving a more colorful and varied selection of foods. Some foods that our children love will probably have to be consumed in smaller amounts, but almost no food will have to be totally eliminated from their meals. A diet designed to lower cancer risk can and should be a diet that is not only healthy and safe but is also tasty, inviting, and fun. What's the best part? By changing our family's meal plans, we positively affect everybody's health.

7

You *Can* Reduce Your Child's Risk of Developing Osteoporosis

Most of us typically believe that osteoporosis is a disease of the elderly. It's true that the disease manifests later in life, but until now, the best-kept secret has been that the roots of this disease begin in childhood when bone growth is optimal. Since osteoporosis is a disease for which no cure exists, making the necessary nutritional and activity changes during infancy, childhood, and adolescence is the only prescription for reducing our children's risk of developing brittle bones later in life.

It's funny how our bodies somehow know more than we do—during each of my pregnancies with my older girls, I craved calcium-laden foods, but didn't know why. I couldn't get enough milk and grilled cheese sandwiches. I now know that the extra calcium probably helped build more bone. Just don't go overboard—it took me a long time to walk off those yummy sandwiches!

The Silent Disease

Osteoporosis, or porous bones, is often called the silent disease because bone loss occurs without symptoms. People may not even know that they have the disease until their bones become so weak that a sudden strain, bump, or fall causes a fracture of the hip, spine, or wrist. It's certainly not a future we want to give to our children.

Yet even though researchers are learning more about this debilitating disease, the osteoporosis epidemic is actually growing in this country. Today, the National Osteoporosis Foundation reports the following:

- Osteoporosis is a major public health threat for twenty-eight million Americans, 80 percent of whom are women.

- One out of every two women and one in eight men over fifty will have an osteoporosis-related fracture in their lifetime.

- Osteoporosis can strike at any age.

- Osteoporosis is responsible for more than 1.5 million fractures annually, including 300,000 hip fractures, and approximately 700,000 vertebral fractures, 250,000 wrist fractures, and more than 300,000 fractures at other sites.

How It Works: Bone is a dynamic tissue. All through life bone tissue is being formed and lost at the same time. Calcium is an integral part of bone tissue, so that as bone is formed more calcium is deposited, and as bone breaks down, more calcium is lost. From fetal life until early adult life, more bone is formed than lost, and more calcium is deposited into bone than is lost from bone. At this time of life, the net change in bone growth is positive, and bones become larger, thicker, and stronger. During the teen years, almost one-half of the adult skeleton is formed.

The ratio of bone loss to bone growth changes for women in their early thirties and men in their early forties. At this time, more bone is lost than is deposited. That means that each day after about 30, a woman loses more bone than she can replace. And at menopause, this ratio changes again, with bone loss increasing and far outstripping the creation of new bone. As bone loss continues to outpace bone growth, osteoporosis may occur. Bones can become thin, weak, and brittle, and finally, a fracture may occur.

In men, the much slower process of bone loss exceeding bone growth is seen from about age 40 throughout the rest of their lives without any dramatic changes. Osteoporosis does occur in men, but much less frequently and less severely than in women. The disease occurs ten times as frequently in women as in men.

Clearly, there are only two ways to prevent osteoporosis: slow down the rate of bone loss, or speed up the rate of bone growth. Increasing the amount of bone growth is best achieved during the period when bone is normally growing faster than it is being lost. The strategy for preventing osteoporosis is to build up such high reserves of bone that they cannot be exhausted even during the long period of bone loss, which comes with certainty in our later years.

For me, this was one of the most amazing findings in this new nutritional research—that we have the capability of storing enough calcium to ensure ourselves strong bones in our later lives. What a powerful bit of knowledge for parents!

The Genetic Connection

We have already seen that girls are ten times more likely to be afflicted with osteoporosis in later life than boys. However, even among girls, the risks may vary.

Our bone structure can present a risk factor. Daughters of large-framed, heavier mothers are at lower risk than are daughters of small, thin mothers.

Race is another genetic factor to consider. Our Caucasian and Asian children are at the highest risk, while our African-American sons and daughters are at lower risk for this disease.

Family medical history counts, too. If you have a family member who has been diagnosed with osteoporosis or a family member who has lost height as they aged, your child is in a high-risk category. It would be wise to inform your pediatrician of your immediate family's medical history.

Dr. W *Medications complicate the picture, as well. Children who have taken, or are currently taking, certain drugs such as cortisone (or corticosteroid) medications must also be considered at higher risk. To a lesser degree, but more relevant in children, prolonged bed rest from any illness can result in poor bone growth. Any girl with any of these risk factors must be considered at high risk for osteoporosis. Any boy with an illness that requires long periods of bed rest or the use of cortisonelike drugs must also be considered at higher risk.*

The Nutrition Connection

During infancy and childhood, a hormonal milieu exists in our bodies that strongly favors bone growth. But for bone growth to reach its maximum potential during this time, certain nutrients must be assimilated into the body. For our children to attain maximum bone growth, they need enough calcium and vitamin D. Without proper nutrition to provide enough of these nutrients, we may be setting them up for osteoporosis later in life.

How It Works: Calcium from our food is absorbed into the blood and then carefully distributed between our bones and other cells. The rate of absorption is controlled by another nutrient, vitamin D, which comes from our foods and from sunlight. While in the liver and kidneys, vitamin D is converted into a hormone that increases sufficient calcium absorption for bone growth. In addition, the form of calcium we take in is just as important as the amount we consume. Calcium is best absorbed from milk and other dairy foods. When that's not possible, calcium supplementation is recommended—calcium citrate is the supplemented form most easily absorbed. You may want to look for calcium chews that are especially formulated for kids.

The rate of calcium absorption is also affected by certain foods. Phosphorus, especially phosphorus-abundant soft drinks, inhibits calcium from reaching our bones. Calcium and phosphorus compete with each other for the same transportation out of our intestines. To get a better picture, think of a railroad train with a limited number of seats, each seat occupied by either a calcium or phosphorus molecule. When more phosphorus molecules are present, fewer seats are available for the calcium molecules. Vitamin D increases calcium absorption by adding more seats to the railroad car. But if more greedy phosphorus (soft drinks) comes into the car, the calcium molecules will be bumped off the train before they can take their seats, denying them transportation to their final destination.

(For a list of calcium-rich foods, please see chapter 9, "Your New Infant.")

The Exercise Connection

If we had to list an activity our school-age children did every day without fail, most of us would probably have to say: "sitting on the couch watching TV," or "sitting in front of a computer chatting with friends." Well, these two activities—or nonactivities, if you will—are exactly the kind of thing that promotes bone loss in our children. Our sedentary sons and daughters are at greater risk for osteoporosis than our more active children. (Remember, we said that inactivity such as prolonged bed rest could affect poor bone growth.)

Keeping our kids active is important; and choosing the right type of activity is also essential. Weight-bearing exercise is what promotes bone growth. Some of the best types of weight-bearing exercise for building strong bones in our children are running, jumping, walking, dancing, gymnastics, soccer, baseball, football, and volleyball. (Swimming is a great cardiovascular exercise, but it doesn't enhance bone growth.) These types of exercise, coupled with good nutrition, will not only help to reduce our children's risk for osteoporosis, they will help to prevent heart disease and obesity as well.

> **The consequence of prolonged weightlessness in space is a dramatic example of the importance of the bones bearing weight. Ever since NASA began its space missions, the agency has kept a vigilant eye on what that has meant to our astronauts' bodies and minds. One of the findings is that astronauts lose considerable bone during a space mission. At present, this is an intensive area of study.**

Dr. W **Should Your Child Be Tested?**

Bone density tests are not routinely used to measure our children's bone growth because we don't want to expose them to too much X-ray radiation.

However, all children take a tumble now and then, often requiring us to have one of their limbs x-rayed. The next time your child takes a fall that brings him to either an emergency room or your doctor's office for an X-ray, ask the radiologist this question: "Are my child's bones calcifying appropriately?" The answer will help you track your child's bone growth.

It's Never Too Early to Reduce Your Child's Risk of Developing Osteoporosis

When should we start banking good bone growth for our children? Before they are born! The need to eat calcium-rich foods begins during pregnancy and continues throughout our children's lives.

Pregnancy is a most important time for preventing osteoporosis in both you and your baby. Since your fetus takes its calcium from your bones, you need to take in enough calcium during your pregnancy to avoid your own risk of developing osteoporosis. By eating calcium-rich foods and taking a calcium supplement, you'll be protecting yourself and your unborn child.

Feeding our sons and daughters a varied diet of dairy products, fruits and vegetables, proteins and whole grains, and keeping them active, will help them to build a large bone reserve that they can draw upon in their adult lives. It's their best defense against a later debilitating life with osteoporosis.

PART II

From Healthy Kids to Healthy Adults— the Right Foods Make a Difference!

8

Pregnancy: Adult Diseases *Can* Start in the Womb

uring these nine months you and your baby have special nutritional needs. Your baby's nourishment comes directly from you, which is why it's vitally important that you get the necessary nutrients to ensure her proper development. During this time our bodies begin a series of hormonal changes that cause fluid retention, emotional ups and downs and, oh yes, those food cravings! As distracting as they are, these signs actually help us to focus our attention on the need to correctly nourish our babies and ourselves.

I remember when I found out that I was pregnant with my first child and suddenly realized that everything I would be consuming would affect not only me, but the baby growing inside me. It's amazing how that realization can alter your eating habits! As a pregnant mother-to-be, you really are, as they say, "eating for two." It's true. New research tells us that the foods we eat while pregnant, and the amount of weight we gain, can lower our soon-to-be-born baby's risk for heart attacks, stroke, diabetes, high blood pressure, obesity, cancer, and osteoporosis. It's that profound. Starting in the womb, sound nutrition will provide lifelong benefits for your child.

How It Works: Beginning with conception, after the fertilized egg is firmly implanted in the wall of the uterus, the placenta is formed, a pipeline that brings food from your bloodstream to the bloodstream of your fetus. Next, your body begins to prepare for the production of breast milk to nurture your infant after birth. As this maternal adaptation is progressing, your body is continually changing. How your body adapts to these changes is important to your pregnancy. Stress, smoking, alcohol, caffeine, carbonated beverages, lack of exercise, and poor nutrition not only create poor maternal adaptation but can also adversely affect your baby's growth and development.

The Placenta—A Hardworking Organ

Early in pregnancy, the volume of blood circulating through your body begins to increase and feed nutrients to your growing uterus, your increasing breast tissue, and your developing placenta. As these tissues expand in size, more and more blood is required. The increase in blood volume and blood flow to the placenta is the first step in the process of forming the fetal lifeline. The blood brings oxygen and nutrients to the fetus and removes carbon dioxide and waste products.

You and your fetus have two separate blood supplies that do not mix. The job of the hardworking placenta is to continuously move all nutrients and oxygen from your blood into the fetal blood supply and remove all waste products, including carbon dioxide, from fetal blood to your blood. The placenta also acts as a specialized factory, producing substances, such as hormones, that are necessary for proper fetal growth and for maintaining the pregnancy.

During early pregnancy, your placenta is growing quickly, developing the complex nutrient transport system necessary to feed your fetus. In the second trimester of your pregnancy, both the placenta and fetus continue to grow at a rapid rate. The placenta is, in a sense, doing double duty, extracting nutrients for its own growth and for the fetus to use for its development.

While your body is undergoing these complex changes, it begins to undergo another series of changes to prepare for lactation after your baby's birth. During this period, fat tissue is stored deep within your body to provide the fuel you will need as lactation proceeds.

The third trimester of your pregnancy is the period of maximum fetal growth. The placenta is now a mature, fully grown, and efficiently functioning organ. As your due date grows closer, your body will continue to deposit more fat, and you'll notice that your breasts are continuing to develop at a much more rapid pace.

Pregnancy isn't complicated, but it does require good nutrition and proper weight gain during the full term to insure the perfect growth and development of your baby. Poor nutrition, even for a short period of time, can lead to less-than-perfect growth and development of your baby, and can create long-term health consequences.

Weight Gain During Pregnancy

While many women worry about gaining too much weight during pregnancy, Dr. Winick says that the real concern is when we don't gain enough. That's because your pregnancy weight gain is directly correlated to your baby's birth weight. Simply stated, if you don't gain sufficient weight, your baby may not grow adequately, or sufficiently, or to full-term weight.

You need to eat enough to support the increased blood volume needed for your uterus and placenta. If you don't, fewer nutrients will be available to your fetus and its growth will be slower. Your fetus will survive, but it won't grow as large as it should.

Ideally, you're striving to eat enough to deliver a baby who weighs at least 6½ to 7½ pounds. (We're talking about full-term deliveries, and not preemies.) It's amazing what an extra half-pound means to your baby's future. The effects of low birth weight can be devastating in later life and may even lead to heart disease, high blood pressure, diabetes, and stroke. Moreover, low birth weight is a major cause of infant mortality in the world today.

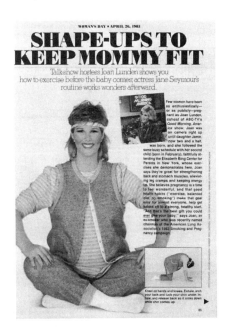

Eight months pregnant during this very uncomfortable shoot, I was reminded of how important it is to exercise during pregnancy.

Your mother or grandmother may not have benefited from the new directives in obstetrics—they were probably told to keep their weight down to avoid the complications of delivery. During the early 1900s when modern obstetrics was still in its infancy, a lot of mothers-to-be were dying in childbirth. When the baby was too large, delivery became more complicated. To address the problem, obstetricians advised pregnant women to keep their weight gain to a minimum so babies would be smaller and thus safer to deliver.

But the weight gain controversy continued over the years even as obstetrics became more sophisticated. Theories with little factual grounding emerged, such as: "It's healthier for the mother to keep her weight down during pregnancy"; "Mothers who gain too much weight are more likely to develop toxemia"; and "Too much weight gain during pregnancy will lead to a permanent weight problem later in life." These theories have circulated for years and have led to a systematic self-imposed reduction in food intake during pregnancy.

Today obstetrics is a highly advanced specialty, and maternal mortality in supervised pregnancies is extremely rare—no matter what the size of the baby. We've now come full circle, and the focus has shifted from the survival of mothers to the optimal weight of babies.

Dr. W *I can't stress enough how very important weight gain is during pregnancy. Several studies, first carried out in England and then confirmed in Sweden and the United States, have demonstrated that babies who were born with a low birth weight showed higher incidences of coronary heart disease, stroke, high blood pressure, high cholesterol, and diabetes than children born with a normal birth weight. Again, to assure that your baby has the best start in life, it's imperative that you gain the proper amount of weight.*

HOW MUCH WEIGHT SHOULD YOU GAIN? If your weight was normal before pregnancy, ideally you should gain twenty-five to thirty pounds: approximately two to five pounds during the first trimester, and three to four pounds per month during the second and third trimesters. If you were underweight before pregnancy, you should gain somewhat more to build up your reserves. If you were overweight, you should gain somewhat less, and if you are considered obese, you should still gain at least fifteen pounds. Pregnancy is not the time to attempt weight reduction.

HOW MANY CALORIES SHOULD YOU CONSUME? Depending on your height and weight, you'll need to consume 300 to 500 extra calories per day to maintain a normal pregnancy—that is, 300 to 500 calories above the normally recommended 2,100 for an adult female. This means that the average pregnant woman should consume at least 2,400 calories a day. These are average figures: your body has ways of dealing with caloric fluctuations—more calories may be consumed on some days, fewer calories on others. But over your entire pregnancy, by just adding a little more food, you'll help to avoid having a low-birth-weight baby.

> ### Here's How Your Pregnancy Weight Adds Up:
> - **The growth of your breasts and uterus adds five to seven pounds.**
> - **The increase in your blood volume adds one to two pounds.**
> - **Fat storage for lactation adds six to eight pounds.**
>
> **Your maternal weight gain contributes twelve to seventeen pounds.**
>
> **Add to this the weight of your fetus, placenta, and amniotic fluid:**
> - **Your fetus adds six and one-half to eight pounds.**
> - **Your placenta adds one to two pounds.**
> - **Your amniotic fluid adds one-half to one pound.**
>
> **Your fetus, placenta, and amniotic fluids contribute another eight to eleven pounds.**
>
> **These two weight factors roughly total twenty to twenty-eight pounds.**

What Nutrients Are Needed During Pregnancy?

For the most part, if you ate a well-balanced diet before becoming pregnant, and you add the additional calories recommended, vitamin and mineral requirements can easily be met. However, there are several nutrients that you should pay special attention to: protein, folic acid, vitamin C, vitamin D, iron, calcium, and zinc.

PROTEIN Your growing fetus requires large amounts of amino acids—the components of protein—in order to build its own tissues. Normally, these amino acids are extracted from your blood by the placenta, but if your diet is low in protein, this extraction may happen at the expense of your own tissue, especially your muscle tissue. Over the course of several pregnancies, especially if your diet between pregnancies has not been high in protein and therefore essential amino acids, your body may become depleted and your fetus may grow poorly.

During pregnancy protein requirements increase to 60 to 75 grams per day. However, most American women consume more than that before becoming pregnant. You'll find protein in red meat, chicken, fish, milk, cheese, yogurts, eggs, beans, lentils, and tofu.

THE VEGETARIAN EXCEPTION There is one exception to this rule, and it applies to those of you who are pure vegetarians (vegans) and eat no meat, fish, fowl, milk products, or eggs. If you are a vegan, you probably know that your diet is potentially low in protein and that care must be taken to ensure consumption of proper nutrients. Vegans need to remember that although grains and legumes both lack some protein elements, eaten together in a diet, they complement each other, providing a complete protein comparable to that in meat, fish, fowl, and eggs. The American Dietetic Association now states that complementary proteins do not need to be consumed at the same time. Consuming various sources over the course of the day should ensure adequacy in healthy individuals. If you're a vegan and become pregnant, you should continue eating the complementary proteins, adding 300 to 500 calories in a balanced form rather than as pure carbohydrate. In addition, since vitamin B_{12} is absent in a vegan diet, you should be taking a B_{12} supplement. If you follow these simple rules, plus the others discussed below, there's no reason to give up your vegan practice when you become pregnant.

More restricted macrobiotic diets should be avoided—they're too low in calories and almost every other essential nutrient—and can be dangerous, even if practiced for only a short time during your pregnancy.

VITAMINS The Nutrients for Pregnancy table outlines the recommended dietary allowance (RDA) for the six nutrients most important during pregnancy, and the best dietary sources of those nutrients.

Nutrients for Pregnancy - RDA

Nutrient	RDA	Best Source
Protein	60 grams	Meat, fish, poultry, eggs, milk, milk products, legumes, and grains
Calcium	1,200 mg	Milk (all forms), yogurt, cheese, leafy green vegetables, clams, oysters, and almonds
Iron	30 mg	Liver, meat, fish, poultry, enriched whole grain cereals and breads, legumes, leafy green vegetables, dried prunes, apricots, raisins, and foods cooked in cast-iron pans
Folic Acid (Should be supplemented)	400 mcg	Liver, yeast, leafy green vegetables, legumes, whole grains, fruits, and vegetables
Pyridoxine (B_6)	2.2 mg	Wheat germ, meat, liver, whole grains, peanuts, soybeans and corn
B_{12}	2.2 mcg	All Meat products, yeast, and tofu

Folic Acid & B Vitamins Certain vitamins tend to be in short supply in our diets but are necessary in greater amounts during pregnancy. These include folic acid (also known as vitamin B_9), vitamin B_{12}, and vitamin B_6. Both folic acid and vitamin B_{12} are particularly necessary in tissues that are undergoing rapid growth. To avoid deficiency symptoms, such as anemia, particular attention should be paid to dietary sources of these vitamins. Vitamin B_{12} is found only in animal products. If you're a strict vegetarian, you must get this vitamin from other dietary sources, or take a supplement. For good dietary sources of folate turn to green leafy vegetables, beans and dried peas, asparagus, citrus fruit, and grain products—cereals and breads—that are now fortified with folic acid.

The evidence is quite conclusive that a deficiency in folic acid during the very early stages of your pregnancy can lead to malformations in the brain and spinal cord of your baby. For that reason, all women contemplating pregnancy should take a folic

Daily Essential Nutrients Food Source

Essential Nutrients	Food Source	Servings Per Day
Protein and Iron	Meat, fish, poultry, eggs, nuts, legumes, and grains	Four
Calcium and Protein	Milk, yogurt, and cheese—regular, low fat, and fat free	Four
Vitamins A and C (Fiber)	All fruits, leafy, red/orange and green vegetables, and potatoes	Five
B Vitamins, Iron (Fiber)	Enriched whole grains—fortified cereals, whole wheat/multi-grain breads, baked goods, and pastas	Four
Water	Water, juice, herbal teas, decaffeinated coffee/tea, fruits, and vegetables	Six to Eight

acid supplement (800 mg) beginning two months before conception and continue it throughout the pregnancy. When health professionals began prescribing folic acid, the incidence of nervous system (spina bifida) defects dropped almost to zero.

Note: If you were taking contraceptive pills several months or more prior to your pregnancy, your supply of folic acid and vitamins B_6 and B_{12} may have been depleted. The pill apparently interferes with the metabolism of these three vitamins. Check with your doctor. She may recommend a supplement.

Iron Iron is so important to expectant mothers that, during the first trimester, our bodies respond by developing a special mechanism in the gastrointestinal tract to absorb this essential mineral. Even if we're consuming large amounts of red meat and liver, our typical daily diet doesn't supply all of the iron we require during pregnancy. Since iron is essential for the production of red blood cells, it is vital to the health of both mother and child. Our iron requirements increase during pregnancy in order to satisfy the mother's increased blood volume demand, as well as supply red blood cells directly to the developing fetus.

Dr. W

In the 1960s, the March of Dimes opened its first birth defects clinic at New York Hospital, and I was its first director. A good friend of mine had been chosen as "Mother of the Year" and later became the spokesperson for the March of Dimes.

Karen, the national poster child from our clinic, was a beautiful five-year-old suffering from spina bifida. She was paralyzed below the base of her spine and walked with braces and crutches. My friend, who was visiting for the announcement and for photographs, walked around, talked to all of the children, played the piano, and sang "Twinkle, Twinkle Little Star" with them. To open her conversation with our poster child, she said, "Do you know that I've known Dr. Winick since I was five years old?" Little Karen looked at her and answered: "So what? I've known him since I was born."

I often think of Karen and the devastating effects spina bifida had on her life. My wish, of course, is that we would have known the benefits of folic acid before she was born. It would have altered her life dramatically.

Most physicians prescribe 30 to 60 mg of iron per day. Iron won't harm either you or your fetus and is strongly recommended during your entire pregnancy. If you don't choose to take a supplement, or if your doctor has determined that your body has sufficient iron stores, you can avoid an iron deficiency by increasing your intake of iron-rich foods. Eat a wide assortment of red meats, chicken, pork, eggs, dried fruit, dark leafy greens, iron fortified breads and cereals, and dried beans and legumes such as navy beans, kidney beans, and lentils.

When selecting your iron-rich food sources, please keep this in mind: iron from meat is better absorbed than iron from plants. But the iron content of a food is only

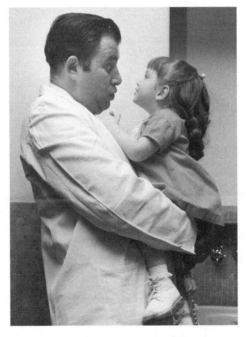

Dr. Winick and Karen, March of Dimes Poster Child

> **TIP**
>
> *A Good Pregnancy Breakfast:*
>
> **A glass of OJ or an orange**
>
> **A bowl of high-fiber fortified cereal—with raisins (use skim or 2% milk)**
>
> **One scrambled or poached egg**
>
> **This meal will provide you with a great amount of vitamin C and readily absorbable iron.**

one consideration. There are other dietary factors that can affect iron absorption. Vitamin C, for example, increases the absorption of iron, so include a vitamin C-rich food with every meal to get the most iron out of the other foods you eat. Look for vitamin C from fresh fruits and vegetables, and freshly squeezed fruit juices and smoothies. On the other hand, certain non-fortified cereals and breads may decrease absorption, which is why you should choose iron-fortified products, whenever possible.

Calcium Calcium is required for bone formation, so increasing your intake of calcium during pregnancy will protect your bones and your baby's growing bones. During pregnancy, although your overall calcium balance may be positive—more comes in than goes out—a significant amount of the incoming calcium must go to the fetus. Calcium absorption during pregnancy is much more efficient than it was prior to pregnancy, nevertheless, if you don't increase your calcium intake, the fetus may very well drain your supply and leave you with a negative calcium balance. In other words, your bones will weaken. More calcium may also be depleted when breast-feeding, and that can cause further stress on your bones. However, by eating calcium-rich foods like milk, yogurt, and cheese, you can come through your pregnancy with a positive calcium balance, and protect yourself against osteoporosis.

If for some reason you're not drinking sufficient milk or eating milk products, then you should take a calcium supplement (500 to 1,000 mg/per day—depending on your intake of milk and dairy products). Be aware that even a prenatal multivitamin does not contain sufficient calcium to meet your increased needs. Since the body always excretes excess calcium, there's no danger in taking a supplement.

It's important to understand that the rate of the absorption of calcium is controlled through the gastrointestinal tract, so what you eat can profoundly influence calcium absorption. Just as foods high in vitamin D, like fish, milk, and yogurt, are needed to help absorb calcium, carbonated soft drinks, with their high phosphorus content, will decrease the amount of calcium absorbed. Unfortunately, because we consume so many carbonated soft drinks, our American diet is extremely high in phosphorus content. To raise your rate of calcium absorption, simply reduce the amount of phosphorus in your diet. It's not difficult to do. Next time you're thirsty, instead of your typical phosphorus-laden soda, reach for a glass of water, natural fruit juice, or a delicious fruit smoothie.

Zinc We now have abundant evidence proving that a zinc deficiency during pregnancy can affect the fetus. Zinc is an essential nutrient particularly needed by rapidly growing tissues. Animal studies have shown that a zinc deficiency during pregnancy results in severe fetal growth retardation and in serious malformations. Human studies have shown that low zinc levels in both amniotic fluid and maternal blood have been associated with cases of poor fetal growth.

Foods rich in zinc are usually rich in iron as well. That's why eating an iron-rich diet is key to protecting you against both iron and zinc deficiencies.

Water and Fluids Water and fluids play a very important role during pregnancy, because they transport the nutrients to your baby via the placenta. So be sure to drink at least six to eight glasses of fluids. Overweight women may require more fluids.

Take A Pregnant Pause

Okay, you've heard it before, but it's vitally important for the health of your baby to honor the big three no-no's—NO smoking, NO alcohol, and NO caffeine. Any one of these may retard fetal growth, which means that your baby could be born with a low birth weight or suffer from fetal malnutrition. Moreover, drinking even the smallest amounts of alcohol may put your baby at risk for fetal alcohol syndrome.

SMOKING Cigarette smoking during pregnancy *will* retard fetal growth. The effect is progressive—as the number of cigarettes smoked increases, the chances of your baby's size increasing becomes ever smaller. While we're not certain exactly why this happens, the best

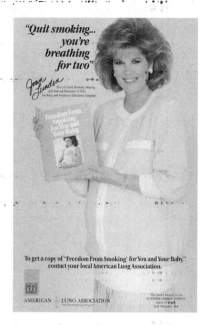

I was eight months pregnant when I shot this poster to remind women of the dangers of smoking while pregnant.

evidence available today suggests that nicotine or other substances in the smoke may cause constriction of the blood vessels feeding the uterus and placenta at the fetal pipeline. Ultimately, the amount of blood reaching the maternal side of the placenta is reduced, which then limits the quantity of nutrients available for the placenta to transport to the fetus.

We also know that smoking reduces the appetite, which means that food intake is reduced. And as we've learned that, in itself, can lead to a lower birth rate for your baby.

The evidence couldn't be clearer. The more you smoke, the greater the chance for a lower birth weight baby. What's the solution? Stop smoking, or at the very least cut way back on cigarette smoking during pregnancy. Even if you cut back significantly during your pregnancy, the evidence suggests that your fetus will benefit. Of course, quitting is the best decision hands-down, but if you feel you can only cut back, the earlier you begin, the better.

Every time I think about pregnant women smoking, I'm reminded of an amazing segment we did several years ago on *Good Morning America*. A woman in her fifth month of pregnancy underwent an ultrasound live on our program. Viewers saw how the tiny unborn baby would recoil each time the woman puffed on a cigarette. When the mother inhaled the nicotine and carbon monoxide, it reached the placenta almost immediately, preventing the fetus from getting oxygen and nutrients. I'll never forget that.

ALCOHOL No alcohol should be consumed during pregnancy. Whether you're a heavy drinker or a social drinker, by consuming *any* alcohol you're putting your baby at risk for fetal alcohol syndrome. This isn't a future you want to offer your child. Fetal alcohol syndrome manifests itself in facial and other physical malformations often associated with mental retardation. The risk isn't determined by how much you drink, but simply by drinking at all. In fact, these abnormalities have been reported in women who drank only small amounts of alcohol. So, please, play it safe. During your pregnancy, drink no alcohol.

CAFFEINE Animal studies and some human studies have shown us that drinking large amounts of caffeine may cause abnormalities in fetal growth. Although the risk of these abnormalities appears to be much smaller than with heavy smoking or alcohol consumption, if you are a very heavy coffee drinker (eight to ten cups per day), it is strongly recommended that you cut down during your pregnancy.

Remember that caffeine is also present in certain drugs and over-the-counter painkillers. A good rule is not to use any drugs during pregnancy without consulting your doctor. If the drug contains caffeine, it should be avoided.

Fish Warning

Exposure to high levels of mercury is unsafe for your unborn child and young children. Pregnant or breast-feeding women, women who may become pregnant, and young children should avoid those fish highest in mercury including: king mackerel, shark, swordfish, and tilefish.

It's okay to eat other fish, especially fatty fish such as herring, mackerel, salmon, sardines and tuna. These fish contain all those wonderful omega 3 fatty acids which are great for your heart, may slow tumor growth, and possibly decrease inflammation. The best advice is to eat a variety of fish twice a week.

(We are concerned, however, about the reports of carcinogens in certain farmed fish, especially salmon. When buying salmon, choose domestic farmed over imported farmed. Wild salmon and canned salmon are even better choices.)

Putting It All Together

Good nutrition is by far the most powerful gift you can offer to your soon-to-be-born baby. Eating a balanced and healthful diet throughout your pregnancy is your goal, but sometimes there are challenges to overcome—you may feel tired and nauseous. But don't skip meals. It's important to eat—and eat well.

One of the nice things about pregnancy is that it's the perfect time to rethink all of your eating habits, and even your relationship with food. This certainly isn't the time to be dieting. Fats are actually very important for you and your developing baby, as are calories. Let your appetite determine the amount you eat. Rather than fighting those food urges, let them help provide the route to proper nutrition. This doesn't mean going crazy with food—it was so hard for me to lose those extra pounds that I gained during each pregnancy—but it does mean following weight-gain recommendations. There isn't a better time to alter any less-than-healthy habits you may have, like cigarette smoking, alcohol and caffeine consumption. Let this be your golden opportunity to clean up your health for your baby, and in the long run, for yourself. By rethinking your food choices and lifestyle habits now, after your baby is born you will have established healthy, new eating patterns that will set the standard in your home for preventing adult diseases.

9

Your New Infant

Nothing in the world can match the thrill of cradling your newborn baby in your arms as you leave the hospital and head for home. Holding your tiny, helpless infant (or infants, as the case may be!), who is completely dependent upon you for his survival, is both exhilarating and daunting. All of your nurturing instincts are awakened and are ready to jump into action. Of course, you're just a little nervous—after all, you want to do everything right.

So many wondrous changes take place every day as your baby begins to grow and become more and more independent. Some are clearly perceptible: babbling to talking, crawling to walking, sucking to chewing, to using a spoon. Others are less visible—every organ in your baby's body will grow and develop in such a way as to be able to carry out its specific job.

One of the first things for you to realize is that your newborn is not a little adult but an immature, helpless creature with the capacity to become an

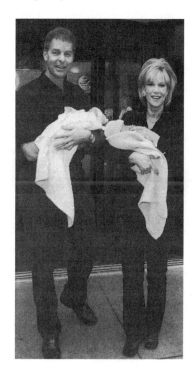

My husband Jeff and I begin our adventure with newborn twins Kate and Max.

adult. We can't expect that tiny body to do things for which he isn't ready. That's why you want to feed your newborn the right nutrients and provide him with the fuel and the building blocks to grow and mature at the proper rate.

The Nutrients Your Baby Needs

Although your newborn is tiny, you might be surprised to learn that he has a much greater requirement for nutrients—fat, protein, carbohydrates—and calories than we do as adults. For example, if you delivered a seven-and-a-half-pound full-term infant, he will require about 60 calories per pound or 390 calories a day. Although 390 calories doesn't sound like a lot, if an adult weighing 154 pounds ate comparably, he'd be taking in over 9,000 calories a day!

Your newborn needs these calories and nutrients to ensure he'll grow and develop normally and that his cells will be properly nourished. A poorly nourished infant will not only grow improperly, but his cellular development may also be impaired. And an overly nourished infant who receives too much of the wrong food will be set up for a lifetime of obesity.

How It Works: In infancy, cells grow and develop at a faster rate than at any other time in life. During the first twelve months, your infant's weight will triple. His developing immune and digestive systems will be almost equal to the immune and digestive systems of an adult. Moreover, by eighteen months of age, all of his brain cells will be fully developed.

Your baby's cells are profoundly affected by early nutrition. His organs will increase in size either by an increase in the *number* of cells or by an enlargement of the *size* of already existing cells.

Deciding Whether to Breast- or Bottle-Feed

New parents are faced with so many decisions—and one of the first is deciding whether to breast-feed or bottle-feed. I don't think anyone will argue that breast milk is not the best milk. It provides the best source of calories and nutrients for your baby. Mother Nature designed breast milk to support the growth of your infant, to adjust to the maturity of your baby's gastrointestinal tract, and to pass on protective antibodies not passed on during pregnancy. Formula manufacturers come close to duplicating it, but they still haven't perfected Mother Nature's handiwork. The quantity and nature of the protein in breast milk has been most difficult to imitate, even in formulas designed to simulate human milk most precisely. Breast milk contains just the right amount of fatty acids, lactose, water, and amino acids for human digestion, brain development, and growth.

Neither choice is wrong, although experts agree that when possible, breast-feeding is preferred. However, you may discover that breast-feeding is not possible or just not right for you. In my case, I breast-fed my three older girls, but not my twins, Kate and Max. They were carried with the help of a gestational surrogate, so I knew I would be bottle-feeding. But it does allow me to speak from having had both experiences. Whatever you choose, I urge you to put away any guilt you may feel. You don't want your new baby to sense your anxiety, especially since either option will do the job.

BREAST-FEEDING More than two decades of research have established that breast-fed infants have lower rates of hospital admissions, ear infections, diarrhea, rashes, allergies, and chronic disease than bottle-fed babies. Studies from the American Academy of Pediatrics have shown that breast-fed babies have fewer illnesses and are protected in varying degrees from pneumonia, botulism, bronchitis, staphylococcal infections,

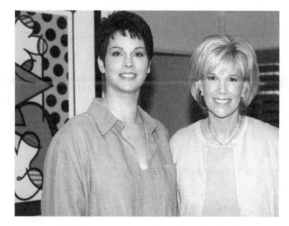

My wonderful surrogate Deborah Bolig had a picture-perfect pregnancy.

influenza, ear infections, and German measles. A recent study from England also concluded that breast-feeding is linked to heart-healthy benefits in adulthood. Early exposure to breast milk as a baby may help to program fat metabolism later in life and produce lower cholesterol levels as an adult. And Dr. Winick would be quick to point out that bottle-fed infants tend to be fatter than breast-fed infants, although not necessarily healthier.

Breast milk offers your baby the vitamins and minerals he needs in the most digestible form. And even though cow's milk contains more calcium, breast milk contains the ideal calcium-to-phosphorus ratio and is better absorbed by your infant's digestive and skeletal systems. Infancy is the perfect time to start building calcium reserves that your child can call upon later in his or her life.

Breast milk also contains a highly absorbable iron. Full-term infants who are entirely breast-fed do not become iron deficient. Breast-fed babies can triple their birth weight in their first year of life and maintain a normal iron status with no iron supplementation. But routine iron supplementation may be appropriate for a premature infant, whose iron stores are low at birth.

How It Works: Breast milk goes through three stages, each designed to correlate with what your baby needs.

First Stage—Colostrum

This first-stage milk is the ideal food for your newborn. It's a thick, sticky, yellowish substance that is high in protein and minerals and contains significant antibodies that protect your infant from illness. This first milk production is limited and causes some moms to worry that their babies aren't getting enough to eat. A word to worried moms—a little goes a long way.

Second Stage—Transitional Milk

On the third or fourth day after delivery, your body begins the second stage of production—transitional milk. This milk appears thinner, but it's actually higher in calories than the colostrum. As the milk volume, fat, and carbohydrate content increases, the number of protective antibodies decreases.

Third Stage—Mature Milk

In the first month, the total quantity of milk produced is about 600 milliliters (ml)—just over a pint—per day. By the sixth month, the milk will increase to about 800 ml (a pint and a half) per day. This mature milk is high in fat and lactose and contains adequate amounts of very high quality protein. Your infant is now ready to receive this richer breast milk and needs no other fluids—even water is unnecessary.

Don't Leave Home Without Them

You can't beat the convenience of breast-feeding. Let me be frank: you always take your breasts with you—you have them wherever you go. I remember when Jamie was seven months old and I had decided to stop breast-feeding. We left on a vacation to the Caribbean, and as we arrived, I found out that the airline had lost my luggage, complete with Jamie's formula. I kicked myself for quitting breast-feeding before the vacation. I had to search the island for the right formula, when I could have just lifted my shirt.

Dr. W

Ellen, a young mother, had just given birth to a healthy baby girl. After I had examined her newborn and assured Ellen that everything with the baby was fine, she told me that since this was her first baby, she'd done a lot of reading, understood the importance of colostrum, and planned to breast-feed. But since she'd learned that colostrum doesn't have the same nutritional characteristics of breast milk, she had a question: "Shouldn't I be supplementing my baby with formula while she's getting the colostrum?" "No," I answered. "During these first few days, your baby doesn't need more nourishment. If she's a little hungry, she'll learn to nurse better, she'll get more colostrum, and most importantly, she'll stimulate you to make more milk and go through the transition from colostrum to mature breast milk more smoothly."

Does My Baby Need Supplements?

Breast-fed babies may need nutritional supplements—especially vitamin D. Breast milk is a poor source of vitamin D, which is why pediatricians will recommend supplementing babies with 400 IU daily, which is available in drop form.

Also, during the first year of life when "baby" teeth are forming and erupting, small quantities of fluoride have been shown to be beneficial to the development of strong teeth. For this reason, the Committee on Nutrition of the American Academy of Pediatrics recommends that infants over the age of six months not exposed to fluoridated water be supplemented with fluoride. Check with your pediatrician or pediatric dentist for an age-appropriate dose.

What Mommy Eats, Baby Eats

The concentration of vitamins and minerals in your breast milk depends to some extent on the state of your own nutrition. If you have a serious vitamin and mineral deficiency, it will show up in your breast milk. For example, if you have an iron deficiency, your baby will receive iron-deficient milk. If you are a strict vegetarian, your baby may be at risk for a vitamin B_{12} deficiency. That's why *your* diet during this time is so very important!

To make the perfect breast milk for your baby, you need to eat three nutritious meals and two healthy snacks daily. You need to eat a variety of foods, and drink 8 to 12 glasses of fluids—milk, juice, soup, or water. Remember to limit your intake of phosphorus laden sodas, because they interfere with calcium absorption. Be sure to eat plenty of citrus fruits for vitamin C and whole-grain or fortified-grain products for the B complex vitamins. Limit foods that are high in sugar as well as those that are high in saturated fats, but be careful not to limit your calorie intake. You'll actually need an extra 500 calories a day beyond what you normally ate as long as you are breast-feeding.

Look for those additional calories in extra servings of chicken, turkey, fish, peanut butter, eggs, cheese, milk, lean beef, nuts, whole grain cereals and breads, tofu or beans, and rice. And when you're adding up those extra calories it will be helpful for you to know that fat contains 9 calories per gram, while protein and carbohydrates contain 4 calories per gram each. Make sure to eat a balance of protein, carbohydrates, and fat, and emphasize foods that are rich in calcium and iron.

CALCIUM To grow good bones and prevent osteoporosis later in life, a good calcium supply is important to you and to your infant. Your best source of calcium can be found in all dairy products—milk, cheese, and yogurt. You can also find good sources in canned salmon and sardines, almonds, collard greens, kale, turnip greens, tofu (processed with calcium), and other soy products. If for some reason your diet doesn't contain enough calcium-rich foods, Dr. Winick recommends taking a calcium supplement.

▶ **TIP** Certain foods you eat may have adverse effects on your baby. For example, spicy foods and cabbage may cause your baby to become gassy and fussy.

Keep a food diary while breast-feeding. If your baby experiences any discomfort, check to see what you ate and eliminate that food from your diet for a while.

This chart shows you foods that provide 300 mg of calcium per serving:

Calcium-Rich Foods
(Each serving provides 300 mg of calcium)

Food	Serving Size
Almonds (chopped)	1 cup
Yogurt	6 to 8 ounces
Cheddar Cheese	1½ ounces
Collard Greens (Frozen—chopped)	1 cup
Cottage Cheese (Regular or Fat Free)	1½ cups
Evaporated Milk (Unsweetened)	4 ounces
Broccoli	1¾ cups
Canned Salmon	4 ounces
Milk (Whole, Low Fat, or Skim)	8 ounces
Turnip Greens (Frozen)	1½ cups

IRON Although the iron in breast milk is in a highly absorbable form and the occurrence of an iron deficiency in breast-fed infants is very rare, your breast milk reflects the iron stores within your body. That's why it's important for you to include iron-rich foods such as beef, chicken, liver, egg yolks, tofu, spinach, lentils, soybeans, and dried apricots, as well as fortified breads and cereals, to your breast-feeding diet.

> **Dr. W**
>
> *Carly had recently given birth to a boy, her first child, who was a normal, beautiful baby, and weighed just under seven pounds. At five feet tall, Carly was overweight before conceiving and after the additional weight she gained during her pregnancy, now wanted to lose at least 50 pounds. She decided to breast-feed but had a question: "Can I breast-feed and diet at the same time without affecting my baby's growth?" It was a terrific question. "Yes," I answered, "but don't lose weight too fast and don't go on any fad diet. Nursing uses up a great deal of energy, which could help you lose some weight," I explained. I did caution her, however, to be sure that her weight loss did not affect her milk production and that her baby continued to be satisfied.*
>
> *Carly chose a balanced diet and was extremely successful with her weight loss. She produced plenty of milk, her baby boy grew normally, and by the time he was a year old, she'd lost 50 pounds.*

CAN MOMMY DIET WHILE BREAST-FEEDING? I know you may want to start losing some of that "baby weight," even while your newborn baby is nursing. Do it slowly! Don't lose more than one pound a week, be sure to eat a balanced diet, and take a multivitamin/multimineral iron-enriched supplement. One important note: do not continue limiting calories if your baby isn't satisfied and isn't gaining weight normally.

CAN MOMMY TAKE MEDICATIONS WHILE BREAST-FEEDING? If you must take a certain medication for health reasons, be sure your pediatrician is alerted. Usually, the medication can be continued, but certain antibiotics, like tetracycline, should be avoided completely while nursing.

Bottle-Feeding

While breast-feeding is recommended, some moms will find that it is simply not an option—or is not right for them. When my daughters Jamie, Lindsay, and Sarah were born, I chose to breast-feed each of them. However, I knew I would be formula-feeding my twins Kate and Max, since my wonderful surrogate, Deborah, carried them. But I wondered whether I would bond with the twins as quickly and powerfully as I had with my older daughters. I'm happy to say it wasn't a matter of breast- or bottle-feeding at all—it was about our private time, our eye contact and physical closeness. And of course, feeding them a food that I knew would help them to grow strong and to flourish.

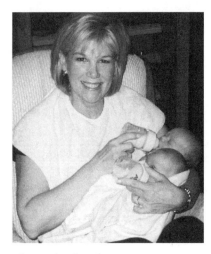

This took a lot of practice.

Formula manufacturers are getting better and better at matching breast milk—constantly reformulating and improving them to keep up with our better understanding of the composition and changes in the real thing. Today's formula products assure adequate levels of vitamins and minerals, and are now offered in different stages that cater to an infant's changing nutritional needs, just like breast milk. So don't worry, your bottle-fed baby will do just fine.

Choosing the Right Formula

There are three kinds of formula: formulas based on cow's milk, which are the most common; soy-based formulas, which contain different proteins and sugars, but the same calories and other nutrients; and a third category referred to as hypoallergenic, for babies who have difficulty digesting soy or cow's milk formulas. Sometimes it takes a little experimenting to see which formula works best for your baby. It's not uncommon for some babies to have a sensitivity to cow's milk formula (any time from two days to four months). Believe me, it won't go unnoticed. After a feeding, your baby may become fretful and cry, even scream. If vomiting occurs and persists (several times in one day), consult your pediatrician—malnutrition and dehydration can rapidly develop. Your pediatrician may recommend changing from cow's milk formula to a soy-based formula—sometimes just for a short period of time.

When my twins were born, I found that my little Kate was an easy baby. She took to the cow's milk formula we gave her without any problems. My little Max wasn't so easy. He really suffered from tummy cramps and flatulence, or as we call it, "tushy talk." After two grueling weeks of long bouts of fussing, followed by bellowing burps and tushy squeaks, we switched his formula to one that was soy based. However, that switch was accompanied by a period of constipation—where we had no good tushy action at all! We made several formula changes, and when it was determined that he was not having a problem with the cow's milk formula, but rather just dealing with an immature digestive tract, he was switched back without too much of a problem. Some babies do have a real sensitivity or allergic reaction to the protein in cow's milk formula. This is less common, but certainly not rare. Your newborn's reaction can manifest as eczema, a troublesome skin rash. Keep your pediatrician informed—she may want to change to a soy-based formula or hypo-allergenic formula.

Dr. W *Studies show that the two fatty acids that are present in breast milk—DHA and ARA— may have a positive influence on a baby's neurological development. While the findings to date are inconclusive, the FDA now allows manufacturers to add DHA and ARA to infant formulas. These new super formulas may be the closest formulas we have to breast milk.*

If you're not feeding your newborn a "super formula," don't worry! Infants grow and develop normally on standard infant formulas. In fact, many hospitals only provide standard formulas. So if your newborn is being fed a standard infant formula, be assured that he is not being deprived.

FOLLOW FORMULA DIRECTIONS CAREFULLY Babies don't come with instructions, but formula does! Whether you choose to use powdered or liquid concentrate, it's important to read labels and follow the directions carefully. Measure the exact amount of water specified in the directions. Underdiluted powder may cause significant problems for your infant (dehydration, kidney problems, etc.) and overdiluted formula will not provide adequate nutrition.

Dr. W

Holly, a new mother, brought her two-week-old baby to see me because she was not thriving. Indeed the child was severely dehydrated, listless, and didn't respond well. Among other questions, I asked Holly what she was feeding her infant. "Infant formula," she told me. When I questioned her further, she said that she was preparing the formula from powder, using two scoops for every one recommended, "to make sure my baby has extra calories," she added. I told Holly that what she was doing was very dangerous. "A child can become very dehydrated," I explained. "Certain important elements in the blood can become too concentrated." Ultimately, Holly's baby responded well to intravenous hydration, and the crisis passed.

My advice: feed your child the amount of powdered formula recommended on the label—no more and no less. Either can be dangerous.

DON'T FORCE YOUR BABY TO EAT When you're bottle-feeding your baby, fight the urge to coax down the last ounce of formula. You may be overfeeding your baby. Bottle-fed infants tend to weigh in heavier at the end of their first year because they are encouraged to finish the bottle. Breast-fed babies aren't urged to "finish the breast." Babies who continue to be overfed tend to be heavier for the rest of their lives. Let your infant determine his or her own level of satisfaction. Don't force that last bit in. Over the course of a year, those little bits add up to a lot of calories.

DON'T GIVE YOUR INFANT MILK All too-often, at around six months of age, many mothers (whether they are bottle-feeding or breast-feeding), wonder if they can change to whole milk. *Don't do it! It is way too early to change to whole milk!* The average six-month-old infant is not mature enough to tolerate it. Your baby should not be given whole milk until she reaches 12 months of age.

Some mothers also wonder if they can wean from the bottle or breast to a fully or partially skimmed milk—perhaps because of recent concern about dietary fat and atherosclerosis, *Again, do not switch to fully or partially skimmed milk—it contains too much protein and not enough fat!* During the first year of life, your baby's kidneys are unable to handle such a load. In addition, the removal of most or all of the fat can lead to an essential fatty-acid deficiency, which can have serious consequences for your baby. So do not feed your baby low fat or skim milk until she is 2 years of age.

Putting It All Together

Whether you breast-feed or formula-feed your newborn, I hope you understand just how important proper nutrition is for both you and your baby. When possible, before making a decision about whether to breast- or bottle-feed, weigh the amazing benefits breast-feeding adds to your baby's health. But in the end, make sure you feel comfortable with your choice. And above all, enjoy this time in your baby's life—they grow up so quickly.

10

Starting Solids

Exactly when is breast milk or formula alone no longer adequate to support your baby's normal growth? It's not always so easy to figure this out, since even the experts don't agree. And sometimes we as parents want to hurry things along and feed our babies solid foods too early. We worry that our babies aren't getting enough to eat, or that they're bored with formula or breast milk, or that their cries are urgent calls for more variety. We also tend to worry that as our babies are growing they're not getting the important nutrients solid foods provide. Well, you can put that worry to bed. In the first months of a baby's life, breast milk or infant formula will supply all the nutrients he needs.

Introducing your baby to solids before he is ready can cause him physical discomfort, promote obesity, and can even trigger lifelong allergies. So, before you rush to introduce your infant to foods other than breast milk or formula, consider how it may affect his lifelong eating patterns, as well as his lifelong health.

Typically, you'll want to introduce your baby to solids when he is between four and six months old and has doubled his birth weight or weighs more than fifteen pounds. Before this time your baby's digestive system isn't prepared to handle any nutrition other than milk. But every child is different. When Max and Kate were almost five-months old they seemed to be hungry all the time and curious about food. I was concerned about starting them on solids too soon, but my husband and I consulted our pediatrician who reassured us that, since the twins were 18 pounds each and consuming so much formula, it was probably time to start them on solids.

Be A Take-Action Parent

Research tells us that adult health problems, including obesity, may begin with the eating patterns we establish as children. So, just as *our* eating habits were determined in part by our parents, it's up to us as take-action parents to realize that our *baby's* eating habits will be influenced by how we feed them. We have a gold mine of research available to us today, so why not take advantage of it? Why not take this time to separate fact from fiction and understand what your baby will need to grow up healthy.

DON'T RUSH SOLIDS Quite often parents start solids too soon because they think that feeding their baby solids will help them sleep through the night. But before you make that mistake, just know that you could be up all night with a very unhappy baby who has a bad tummyache because he couldn't handle the solids.

Dr. W *Years ago a big myth circulated. It went like this . . . Children who eat solid foods earlier develop more rapidly than children who remain on formula or breast milk only. The child who eats a wide variety of foods is thought to be more advanced, the "first kid on the block" to take solid foods. It was a powerful idea, leading many pediatricians to capitulate to parental pleas. These pediatricians reasoned that while early feeding of solid foods wasn't necessary, it could certainly do no harm. And if introducing solid foods early satisfied the parents' needs, it was actually doing some good.*

Today, most pediatricians put their focus on educating parents on the importance of proper nutrition, starting with when and how to introduce solid foods, and which should come first.

UNDERSTAND YOUR BABY'S READINESS CUES As your baby approaches that six month milestone, he will begin to sit up and his head movements will become more controlled. Around this time your baby's tongue thrust reflex will have subsided, and he will have stopped pushing things out of his mouth and started taking them in. It's also likely that he'll have a real curiosity about your eating, and will follow the fork to your mouth with his eyes, or even reach out to grab your food and your spoon! These are baby readiness cues and they're the best signal you'll have that your baby is ready for solid foods.

RESPECT YOUR BABY'S SIGNALS Once you begin offering solid foods, learn to respect your baby's signals. For example, when you bring the spoon to her mouth and she opens her lips, it means she's hungry. And when she closes her lips and turns her head away, it means she doesn't want any more. When Max is hungry

> **TIP** "Suck-suck—swallow." Until your baby reaches four months of age, these are the operative words. She cannot chew and is just learning to swallow. Make sure that your baby's foods are finely pureed and are compatible with her age and digestive abilities. As her skills increase offer foods with more texture and consistency. To start creating proper eating habits and strengthen gums and budding teeth, encourage your baby to chew.

he looks like a little baby bird. The moment I dip the spoon in his food, he opens his mouth and tips his head up! And believe me . . . when he's full, he closes those lips tight. That's my signal. It doesn't matter whether half the jar is left or not. Max has told me that he's full and I need to respect that.

It's important not to try to continue to put food in your baby's mouth, because sometimes he'll eat just to please you. On the other hand, don't be too quick to put the jar away either. Sometimes your baby will just need a moment "to dine," a little breathing room between mouthfuls. Babies understand intuitively that they should eat when they're hungry and stop when they're full, so give your baby a chance to tell you what he needs.

INTRODUCE NEW FOODS ONE AT A TIME One food at a time is the rule for introducing new foods. And make sure that each new food is introduced as a single ingredient. Keep your baby on each new food for at least five days before introducing the next. In this way, if your baby has a sensitivity to something, you'll be able to identify it easily and remove it

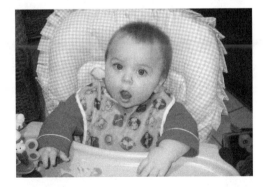

He may look like a little bird . . . but he doesn't eat like one.

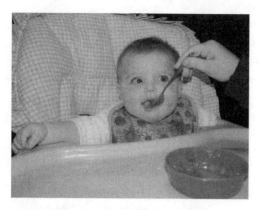

Kate isn't so sure what this solid food thing is all about yet.

from his diet. You can always try to reintroduce that same food a couple of months later to see if your child may be better able to tolerate it.

Start with small-size servings—one or two teaspoons—and gradually increase the serving to three or four teaspoons. This method will allow your baby to experience new food without being overwhelmed. It will also give him time to practice swallowing with smaller amounts of food.

DON'T PASS ALONG YOUR FOOD PREJUDICES Everyone has their own likes and dislikes when it comes to food, but it's important to encourage your baby to be adventurous and to try new foods without a fuss. Try to avoid expressing your own dislikes. Babies remember those funny faces you make, and if your face indicates a dislike of blueberries, well, chances are your baby won't like them either.

Which Foods Come First

Cereals The American Academy of Pediatrics recommends starting with a single-grain, iron-fortified cereal made from rice. This is a good first choice because it is easy to digest, is fortified with iron, and is least likely to cause allergies. You can introduce barley or oatmeal next, but remember to wait five days before the introduction. After your baby has tried all the single-grain cereals, offer her mixed-grain cereals. Rice cereal is available in jars, as a dry mix, or you can make your own by cooking and pureeing rice in a food processor. Just make sure *not* to add any condiments. If you choose the dry mix, follow the directions and keep the consistency fairly liquid by mixing with breast milk, formula, or water. As your baby gets older, the cereal can be mixed into a thicker consistency. Mix

> **Dr. W** *Although most pediatricians recommend iron-enriched cereal as the first solid food, we have no evidence that one food sequence is better than another. Vegetables and fruits may be a better first-food choice—the earlier you introduce your baby to the taste delights of vegetables and fruits, the earlier he will learn to relish them and develop a lifelong love affair with them.*

the cereal in a bowl—not in the baby's bottle—and feed it to him with a spoon. In this way, you'll be encouraging your child to chew and control the intake of excess calories.

One interesting note: some pediatric nutritionists feel that it's so important to establish vegetable and fruit preferences early on, they recommend starting our babies on them even before cereal.

Vegetables and Fruits Whether or not you begin with cereal, you should always start your baby on vegetables before fruits. Introducing the natural taste of vegetables before she's tasted the sweetness of fruit will help her to become a vegetable aficionado. Offer your baby a wide variety—peas, green beans, squash, sweet potatoes, potatoes, and carrots, then introduce strained bananas, peaches, apricots, apples, plums, and pears one by one. Later on, when your baby begins to drink from a cup, you'll be able to offer her natural fruit juice in addition to water. Just make sure you limit the juice to four ounces a day. Excessive intake of fruit juice can decrease her appetite for other nutrient- and energy-rich foods. Moreover, recent studies have shown a direct link between excessive consumption of fruit juice and obesity.

> **Dr. W** *It's a good idea to make complex carbohydrates—whole grains, vegetables, and fruits—a staple in your baby's repertoire early on. These fiber-rich foods are important in preventing cancer and heart disease later in life.*

Protein At about eight or nine months of age, you can introduce your baby to soft egg yolks (hold off on whites until your baby is a year old—they may cause an allergic reaction), strained beef, poultry, veal, pork, beans, and lentils. Cottage cheese and yogurt can also be offered. Proteins may be difficult for your baby to digest, though, so go slowly when introducing them. And understand that not all proteins are suitable to your younger toddler. Peanut butter should be avoided until age two, as should shellfish. Introducing these foods before your baby's second birthday may cause allergies.

If your baby will be following a vegetarian diet, be sure to include complete proteins. In addition to formula or breast milk you can offer cheese and yogurt which contain all the essential amino acids he needs. Vegetable proteins, found in grains (wheat, rice, barley, oats), and legumes (beans, lentils, soybeans, tofu, dried peas) are incomplete (missing one or more essential amino acids). When vegetable proteins are eaten in combination at the same meal, i.e. beans and rice, or separately throughout the day, your baby will receive all the important amino acids she needs.

Note: Nuts and seeds are also a source of incomplete protein for vegetarians, but should not be offered until your child is two years or older.

ADDING TABLE FOODS At about nine to twelve months, your baby can enjoy food from the family table. Gradually she will move from pureed meats to ground meats, and then to finely chopped meats. In addition, she'll probably like rice, potatoes, pasta—or cheese slices and grilled cheese sandwiches. Adult foods can be mashed or cut into bite-sized portions. But don't forget that most of the foods on the table have already been seasoned to accommodate adult tastes. And remember: As more and more table foods are intro-

Dr. W *Babies need healthy fats! Our concern with fat, cholesterol, obesity, and heart disease may lead many parents to limit egg yolks, dairy products, and fatty meats in their children's diets. But this isn't the right time to put your baby on a restrictive diet. Your child is growing rapidly and needs sufficient amounts of essential fatty acids, so provide enough variety to insure that your baby is getting enough healthy fats and don't start him on skim milk until he is two years of age.*

duced, try to avoid high-calorie, high-fat, high-salt, and highly sugared foods. Watch out for using too many processed foods. Choose frozen and fresh whenever possible.

UNDERSTAND THAT SOME FOODS ARE JUST NO-NO'S! Until your baby's first birthday, a number of foods are just not appropriate. Some may cause allergic reactions, and some are just too hard to digest. These foods include egg whites, ice cream, seafood, chocolate, citrus fruits, tomatoes, cucumbers, onions, cabbage, broccoli, spinach, and beets. The Committee on Nutrition of the American Academy of Pediatrics recommends that honey must be avoided during that crucial first year. It contains botulism spores that can cause life-threatening problems for your infant's digestive system. Other foods pose choking hazards. Avoid raisins, grapes, nuts, peanut butter, pieces of hot dogs, and raw carrots.

Commercial or Homemade?

COMMERCIAL BABY FOODS From the 1940s until the 1980s, almost all babies were being fed commercial infant foods. The success of these baby foods was due in no small part to the fact that they were nutritious, well prepared, good tasting, and convenient to use. And it's still true today.

At the same time, however, as more and more combinations of foods were being developed, many were being prepared to suit parental tastes—with salt and sugar added. But as we all became better educated, the baby food industry began catering to infants' tastes instead of our tastes, and now baby foods no longer contain added salt or sugar.

Commercially prepared baby foods have certain advantages: they're carefully prepared with good nutrition in mind. (Nutrients removed in processing, such as vitamins in rice

> ▶ TIP **Never feed your child directly from the baby food jar unless you're sure he'll finish it. When you put a spoon from your baby's mouth straight into the container, you're transferring bacteria from your child's mouth to the jar. When you reseal the jar, you've created a germ-growing environment. The next time you feed your baby, you run the risk of giving him food poisoning.**

cereal, are replaced in the final product.) They're of a consistency that's well tolerated by infants; they're convenient to use; and they're carefully packaged to avoid contamination.

Be aware that some packaged baby foods are super-sized, which makes overfeeding a problem and increases your baby's risk of becoming obese. If you are using commercial baby foods, remember there is "nothing sacred" in the size of the jar. This is not the time to encourage your baby to finish the jar or to "clean her plate." Just keep in mind that as each new food is introduced, a significant amount of the contents may have to be discarded. (Don't store leftovers in the refrigerator for longer than 24 hours.)

HOMEMADE FOODS Given that there is a trend today toward natural foods, a lot of parents are whipping up homemade baby foods. With the aid of a food processor, blender, or food mill, they're pureeing infant foods and storing them in the freezer. Preparing baby foods at home can be less expensive, and it does allow parents to oversee ingredients and control portion size. Before you make your first batch of baby food, buy a jar of commercial baby food so that you can get an idea of the desired consistency.

> **TIP** Try freezing homemade baby food in ice cube trays. A "cube" is equivalent to the serving size a child needs between the ages of six and ten months. If, however, you freeze larger quantities of baby foods, don't refreeze it once it has been defrosted. What isn't consumed at one feeding should be stored in the refrigerator for only a few hours.

Baby food manufacturers have put many years (and many dollars!) into determining the best food for the age and stage of your child, so why not take advantage of all their research! Finally, if you choose to prepare your child's food, don't add salt or sugar, and remember, most canned foods, such as canned peas or green beans, contain salt. Read the label and *if salt has been added, do not feed the product to your baby.* In fact, it's best to select fresh or naturally frozen fruits and vegetables almost exclusively when making your own baby foods.

Baby Steps With Baby's Foods

DON'T SEASON YOUR BABY'S FOOD Before you even think of adding salt or spices to your baby's food, think again. Babies actually like bland foods. In almost all cases, your infant will accept food without any added seasoning, and that includes salt. Remember: Foods that seem bland to us often taste delicious to our infants. And if your family is hooked on salt, this might be a good time for all of you to make some seasoning shifts. Babies mimic family members and many adults salt everything in sight before even tasting it. Give your baby a head start—don't impose your acquired taste for salt on him. Help him avoid a future of high blood pressure and heart disease. The best part is that you'll be helping everyone in your family!

BABIES ARE SWEET ENOUGH WITHOUT SUGAR! Although children are born with a taste for sugar, it would be wise to avoid presweetened foods as much as possible. Read labels for hidden sugars. Offer sweet fruits—homemade applesauce, fruit and Jell-O parfaits, frozen banana treats, or frozen juice pops. Of course, when cooking and baking, certain recipes call for sugar. You might try substituting sweet fruits like pureed apples and dates. And when you do add sugar, try to use it judiciously.

AVOID JUICE When you go to the supermarket, the juices are right next to the baby food jars, so there's a natural tendency to buy juice. But this is not the stage to introduce juices (unless your doctor has specifically recommended it in case of your baby's constipation). Juices are a concentrated source of calories and your baby will already be getting all the vitamins and minerals she needs from the fruits and other foods you will be feeding her.

BE CAUTIOUS WITH TEETHING FOODS Typically, infants start teething by around six or seven months of age. Some pediatricians advocate no teething foods—suggesting that babies teeth on teethers and that parents save crackers and biscuits for mealtimes. If you choose to offer your baby some basic finger foods to provide comfort while those teeth are erupting, be careful to select teething biscuits, sturdy crackers, and bagels. (I buy mini bagels and freeze them before serving to Max and Kate.) But be very cautious. To avoid the risk of choking, *never* leave your baby alone when he's eating teething foods.

Knowing When To Wean

Once your baby is consuming a wide variety of solid foods, it's time to reduce the intake of breast milk or infant formula and begin the weaning process. It's important initially to introduce solid foods as a supplement to breast- or bottle-feeding to insure that your child gets adequate nutrients. After a time, when your baby is eating many different solid foods, he will be getting most of the important nutrients from these new foods.

Your breast-fed infant will respond to the weaning call naturally, gradually cutting back on the intake of breast milk. Your formula-fed infant may need assistance with the process. If your baby is still taking formula from a bottle, to insure that you don't overfeed him, it's generally recommended to keep his intake at around four 6-ounce bottles, or three 8-ounce bottles per day. This will depend on the size of your baby, and also the amount of solid food he is taking. If your baby is drinking from a glass, three 8-ounce glasses per day are enough.

After his first birthday, you can offer either formula or whole milk. As more and more solid foods are being consumed, the amount of milk or formula will be reduced. By the time your baby has been fully weaned, most nutrients will be coming from solid foods, supplemented by the nutrients from milk or formula (about 24 ounces per day).

As the quantity of milk is further reduced, make sure that your baby is given adequate amounts of protein. It can be derived from many sources—meat, dairy products, eggs, fish, and certain vegetables, such as legumes and beans. By offering a variety of these foods, you can be sure that your baby will be getting plenty of protein.

By age two, both breast- and bottle-feeding can be stopped entirely for you will have a fully-fledged toddler on your hands!

 After your child is weaned, if she's consuming a variety of solid foods, she won't need vitamin or mineral supplementation.

Putting It All Together

As parents, we all want our children to be the first to walk, talk . . . and maybe even run for president! We revel in bragging rights, such as, "My child did it first." But when it comes to your child's nutrition, patience is the operative word. This is one of those times when you don't want to rush things.

This can be a happy social time for you and your baby, and a new, healthy eating adventure for everyone. Each day you'll discover more about your baby and he'll discover more about you! Revel in this time of amazement and watch as a world of taste, color, odors, and textures opens up for him. Each new food discovery he makes is an exciting experience. Make it a family affair!

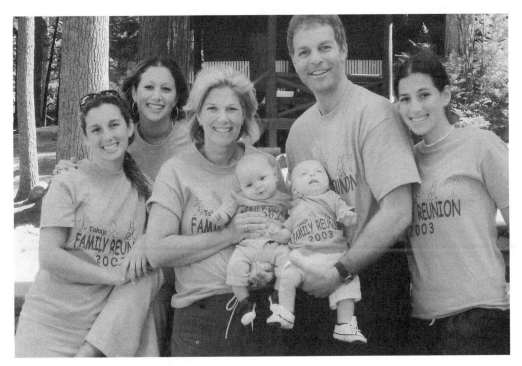

A happy family reunion.

11

Teaching Your Toddler to Thrive

Any parent will tell you that getting a toddler to sit still is not an easy task. But getting your toddler to sit *and* eat a balanced meal can be like swimming upstream in molasses! During these formative years—from the time they begin to "toddle" to almost four years—children are much like sponges, absorbing all the sights, sounds, and tastes in their new world. They're cute, lovable, funny—and since their new favorite word is "No!" they can be exasperating too. Toddlers can be especially trying when their parents are struggling to help them develop positive attitudes toward healthy foods. But, believe me, it's worth all the trouble.

It's important to remember that your child's growth slows down during his second year. While babies usually triple their weight by the time they become toddlers, after that their growth slows down dramatically, so they're not as hungry as they were when they were infants. Parents often worry when their toddler begins to eat less and they don't see the growth they've come to expect. But stop worrying! Toddlers don't actually need as much food as we might think.

Encouraging your toddler to eat too much food can encourage bad eating habits and may set him up for the development of childhood obesity. And of course we now know all too well that adult obesity often has its roots in childhood eating habits, and that the kind of adult obesity that begins in childhood is the most severe and the most difficult to control. That's why the earlier we implement healthy eating habits, the better chance we have of reducing our child's risk not only for obesity, but for Type II diabetes, heart disease, high blood pressure, cancer, and osteoporosis as well. And what parent wouldn't want that?

Be a Take-Action Parent

As parents we need to know what to expect from our toddlers. They are changing both physically and developmentally. They need less food and more independence. You can expect your toddler to be sassy, opinionated, and . . . oh yes, picky. As parents we need to lighten up a little and be less emotional about their eating. We don't want to get into food fights with our toddler, and we don't want to turn the dinner table into a battlefield. Children shouldn't dread mealtime. If we constantly nag our toddler to eat, he may just eat to please us and to get our approval—or simply to get us to stop nagging—and may become an overeater. We want our toddler to learn to eat when he's hungry and stop when he's full. We don't want him to think of food as a punishment or a reward. And we want him to eat the same foods as the rest of the family. How do we accomplish this? Every family is unique. There is no one magical road map to follow. But by adopting some good nutritional guidelines and adapting them to your family's preferences, everyday healthy eating can become an indelible way of life.

RESPECT YOUR TODDLER'S INDEPENDENCE "No-no-no-no-no!" "It's yucky!" "I don't want that new stuff!" "It tastes *funny!*" Your toddler is striving for independence. It's what she's supposed to do at this age. You didn't count on toddler rebellion, but here it is, and you've got your work cut out for you. Yet despite all the protests, this is actually the time in your child's life when you have the most control over her food selections. It just takes patience and perseverance. Oh, and did I mention a good sense of humor?

MAKE EATING FUN As adults, we know that eating is one of life's pleasures, but our toddlers may be more intrigued by the spoons, forks, and plates they can knock to the floor. Every parent knows that game. This is not the time to teach table manners; it's the time to relinquish a little bit of control. Toddlers want to taste and touch everything. That's how they learn. So you're going to have to let your toddler put her hands in her food and try to laugh at it. This is the time to take advantage of your toddler's curiosity and create an interest in food. Remember, messiness is only a problem for parents—not for toddlers!

Treat food as an adventure for both of you, and expose your child to new flavors, new foods, and new cooking methods. Invite your toddler into the kitchen to help you—always supervised, of course! Children are usually more willing to eat any food they've helped prepare. Getting your toddler involved is the best way I know to turn him into a healthy food lover. Here are some ideas to get you started on your adventure.

- Let them be little chefs—wash lettuce, break up veggies.

- Involve them in setting the table and wiping up.

- Make up silly-named menus and create funny names for dishes, and don't forget the jokes! *What did the tablecloth say to the table? Don't move—I've got you covered!*

- Offer colorful, multitextured foods in all the food groups.

- Be creative! Make funny faces on food and whimsical-shaped sandwiches.

- Have a picnic! Throw a blanket down on the living room floor or in the middle of the kitchen floor. You can even pack a basket.

- Mix it up a little bit. Serve breakfast foods for dinner and dinner foods for lunch.

DO AWAY WITH THE CLEAN PLATE RULE Toddlers only eat when they're hungry. And they have tiny stomachs so they eat small portions. They don't eat three meals a day—that was designed to accommodate an adult work schedule—and they shouldn't be expected to clean their plates. Does the idea of cleaning your plate hit close to home? If it does, you're not alone. The clean-your-plate concept probably began after the Great Depression and has continued in most American households. However, today experts stress that it's important that children not feel compelled to clean their plates or even to take those last two bites. They urge parents to break that habit, rethink those old behaviors, and help our children avoid the obesity trap.

BE PATIENT WITH FOOD JAGS Toddlers have entered a stage of separation, and often assert their personalities by expressing their likes and dislikes at the dinner table. They like to feel in charge. And they like to feed themselves too. It's also quite normal when they eat only Cheerios for breakfast, lunch, and dinner for three days straight, and then want only grilled cheese sandwiches. That's called a food jag, a short-term eating habit in which your toddler demands the same food over and over again. Your toddler may choose a favorite food one week and ignore it the next. Don't worry. Continue to offer other foods, but don't make too big a deal of it. This won't last.

DON'T USE FOOD AS A REWARD OR PUNISHMENT Bad behavior should never mean going to bed without dessert, or worse, going to bed without dinner. At the same time, offering food as a reward for good behavior can lay the groundwork for an emotional attachment to certain foods and the need for those foods during times of stress. Of course, the big problem with offering food as a reward is childhood obesity—and we want to do everything we can to prevent that.

DON'T FORCE FOODS Don't worry too much when your toddler doesn't want to eat. If she refuses food, don't force the issue. She'll eat when she's hungry. As a parent, it's important to try to remain calm, and not to scold your child if she spits food out, drops it on the floor, or like many children, secretly feeds it to the dog.

EXPERIMENT WITH NEW FOODS Dr. Winick encourages us to provide our children with a variety of foods, but he also reminds us that introducing new tastes to our toddlers can require some perseverance on our part. When you're experimenting with a new food, it's a good idea to offer your toddler one of his favorites along with the unfamiliar food. Don't try to hide the new food in stews, casseroles, or under gravies. You want your child to trust you. It may take several attempts before your toddler is even willing to taste a particular new food, but keep on trying. I've always found that if you put a little bit on your own plate, your toddler will be more likely to try it. Sometimes it's just a matter of time. Your toddler may reject something one week, but happily try it the next. The important thing, though, is not to give up. If you never serve that food again your toddler could assume that this is a food she will not be expected to eat.

ENCOURAGE A POSITIVE ATTITUDE TOWARD ALL FOODS No food is inherently bad. Not even fat, salt, or sugar. And no one should feel guilty about enjoying a treat from time to time. So if your kids love French fries, indulge them occasionally, but teach them that these treats must be balanced with nutritious foods and eaten in moderation so that they can enjoy them without guilt.

As Greenwich, Connecticut-based clinical nutritionist, Liz Shaio, puts it, "Look at foods in a nonjudgmental way. You're not good if you eat a salad or bad if you have a cookie. What you eat does not define you. Parents need to avoid saying 'I was so good—I only had a salad for lunch,' or 'I was so bad—I ate ice cream last night.' Toddlers pick up on these comments. Madison, a five-year-old girl, recently told me, 'It's good to avoid carbs.' 'What are carbs?' I asked. 'You know, bagels and pasta.' 'Are any carbs good to eat?' I continued. 'Well,' she stumbled, 'I'm not really sure.' I told Madison that in fact she didn't have to avoid carbs. I explained that they are just one of the food groups that we select from every day which our body needs in order to have energy and work properly." I hope she understood.

Dr. W Avoid the Obesity Trap

It's worth repeating. Childhood obesity is an extremely serious problem. Each day new cells, including fat cells, are being added to your toddler's body. It's imperative that we help our children avoid developing too many fat cells. Please remember—once a fat cell forms, it will remain for life! Fat cells may enlarge or shrink, but once formed, they will never disappear. Your toddler will never be able to rid herself of those cells. If she does develop too many fat cells and becomes obese at the age of four or older, she has an 80 percent chance of becoming an obese adult. And it's so much more difficult to treat an obese adult who was an obese child, than to treat an adult who became obese in her adult years. Childhood is a crucial time for preventing your child from accumulating too many dangerous fat cells.

How to Count Calories

So, how many calories should your toddler be getting each day? One to 3 year olds need approximately 1300 calories a day, or 45 calories per pound. Four to six year olds need approximately 1800 calories a day, or 40 calories per pound. But not all calories are created equal, and all too soon you're going to figure out which high-calorie foods your toddler loves to eat. However don't forbid foods completely. Simply cutting back on high-calorie foods and replacing them with foods lower in calories and higher in fiber is a painless way to create good eating habits, and to control weight gain. For instance substituting an 80-calorie apple for a 175-calorie ice-cream cone will save at least 75 calories. It will also provide more of the essential nutrients your child needs.

Do what works best for your family and experiment with alternative cooking methods for your favorite foods. Here are two healthy recipe makeovers to get you started.

Joan's Fat-Free French Fries

Ingredients

> **3 baking potatoes (about 2 pounds) scrubbed**
>
> **Nonstick olive oil or vegetable oil spray**

Directions:

1. Preheat oven to 350 degrees Fahrenheit.

2. Cut potatoes into French fry–sized pieces—about ⅓ inch thick and 1½ to 2 inches long.

3. Spray a sheet pan with nonstick olive oil spray, arrange the potato sticks in one layer and bake for 20 minutes.

4. Put under a broiler until crispy and golden, turning several times.

Rather than salting the fries, try flavoring with other herbs such as rosemary.

Joan's Sweet Potato Oven Fries*

Ingredients

> 2 medium sweet potatoes (1¼ to 1½ pounds) scrubbed
>
> Nonstick vegetable oil spray

Optional Seasoning:

> Mix equal parts ground nutmeg and cinnamon
>
> Mix ⅛ teaspoon each: paprika, garlic flakes, and a pinch of cayenne pepper.

Directions

1. Preheat oven to 400 degrees Fahrenheit.

2. Cut the potatoes crosswise, ¾ inch thick

3. Spray a baking sheet with the nonstick vegetable spray and arrange in one layer.

4. Bake in preheated oven for 15 minutes, then turn them and bake for an additional 10 minutes or until just golden.

5. Top with optional seasonings—or create your own.

* Sweet potatoes are a great source of vitamin A. This recipe provides a great way to get in some vitamin A, and introduce your picky toddler to the joy of sweet potatoes.

Track Your Toddler's Growth

While we don't want to be overly vigilant about our toddler's calorie intake or judgmental with regard to food, Dr. Winick reminds us that we do need to be vigilant about tracking our child's growth. Remember: the overweight child who goes on to become an obese teenager and adult will be at increased risk for coronary artery disease, high blood pressure, diabetes,

> ▶ TIP **Most children will grow about two inches, and gain about four to seven pounds a year.**

and a shorter life. That's why monitoring your child's growth is critical in stopping child-hood obesity in its tracks.

Use the age and gender-appropriate growth charts in this book as a guide. If you notice a sudden surge in the slope of your child's weight line, and little or no change in his height line, you need to take action. Dr. Winick does not recommend putting your toddler on a restrictive diet, but does encourage you to make some significant meal alterations. You can substitute ingredients that are lower in fat. You can change the cooking method, i.e., "oven frying" chicken. You can replace sugary snacks with health-ier treats. In this way, your toddler will gain weight *more slowly* as she grows, and over time will return to the normal weight range for her age and height.

Melissa, an advertising copywriter, was diligent about planning her family's meals, especially those of her three-year-old toddler, Lisa. Although Melissa's pediatrician had told her that Lisa was in the seventy-fifth percentile, which was fine for her age and bone structure, Melissa didn't notice that Lisa had gradually crept up into the eightieth percentile. "I don't know how this could have happened," Melissa told me. I asked her if she knew what snacks and other foods Lisa was eating while at day care. Melissa wasn't sure, but she made it her business to find out.

A few days later, she called me. "The children are eating three snacks a day—one fruit, one ice cream, and one milk and cookies," she said. "Is this why Lisa's gaining weight?"

"Definitely," I told her. "This is a potential obesity problem for all of the children, not just Lisa." I suggested that she speak with the day care providers and recommend that in place of ice cream they provide low-fat frozen yogurt or sorbet, substitute another fruit for the cookies, and serve 1 percent or skim milk instead of whole milk.

Melissa worked with her day care providers to set up a healthy snack program. None of the children, including Lisa, noticed the substitutions—no complaints. By making this small change, Melissa was able to guide Lisa back to the seventy-fifth percentile and possibly avert a lifelong obesity problem.

One important note: Lisa never lost weight, she simply gained more slowly than before. By making minor snack modifications and allowing her weight to catch up with her height, she "grew up and out" of her tendency for obesity.

As soon as the growth line returns to your toddler's normal percentile, you'll know you've saved your child from a serious problem later in life. If your toddler's weight continues to increase, in spite of your best efforts, consult your pediatrician. *Don't wait until your child becomes obese!* It's much more difficult to treat these increased fat cells later on.

What Your Toddler Needs to Grow Up Healthy

CALCIUM To build and support your toddler's growing bones, she needs two servings from the milk group each day. One serving equals one cup of milk or yogurt, or one and one-half ounces of cheese. Another bone-friendly calcium source is canned salmon with the bone. Dr. Winick also points to soup stocks, which, he says, can be very rich in calcium if they're made from meat or fowl with the bones not removed during cooking.

> ▶ TIP **Slip some nonfat dry milk into foods like hot cereals, mashed potatoes, soups, meatballs, and homemade baked goods. Or whip together in a blender a banana with milk and a dash of vanilla for a healthy, tasty shake. Give it a fancier name, like a Vanilla Swirl or a Banana Boogie.**

In the early nineteenth century, a serious problem developed at the London Zoo, which at that time was the largest and most complete zoo in the world. The tigers were developing brittle bones—many suffered from fractures that were healing poorly, and some died of what was being called this "strange disease." The curator visited the zoo in Dublin to see if the same problem was occurring. It wasn't. The reason for the difference? Diet. In London, as part of what they considered a better diet, the bones were removed before the meat or chicken was fed to the animals. As a result, a major source of calcium was removed from their diets, and the tigers developed osteoporosis.

PROTEIN How much protein should your toddler be eating? From one to three years old, 16 grams per day. From four to six years old, 24 grams per day. For example: 1 tablespoon of peanut butter has 4 grams of protein; 1 8 oz glass of milk has 8 grams of protein; and 1 ounce of cheese has 7 grams of protein.

Your toddler may want to live on chicken fingers, but this is a good time to introduce her to other sources of protein, like fish. Naturally low in saturated fat, high in omega-3 fatty acids and protein, fish is a natural for your little one. But can you get him to eat it? Yes, definitely. Toddlers prefer soft, mild-flavored white fish, like cod, catfish, halibut, flounder, and sole. And later they can also become hooked on other seafood such as shrimp, scallops, lobster, and crab. Just look out for hidden fats in packaged, breaded fish sticks.

IRON In the first year of your child's life he will get iron from breast milk, formula, and iron-fortified infant cereals. Now that you've got a toddler on your hands, and he's eating more table food—and fewer fortified foods—you have to make certain he's getting adequate iron. Chicken, beef, spinach, and fortified breakfast cereals (unsweetened) will provide iron support.

FIBER Remember when our mothers told us to eat "roughage"? They were referring to healthy fiber, which influences the digestive system, helps to regulate the bowels, and protects against the development of many diseases, including obesity. To increase the fiber in your toddler's diet, give him more fresh fruits (with skins) and vegetables, whole grains, dried beans, lentils, salads, and nuts.

DON'T FORGET THE FLUIDS Now that your toddler is on the run—if you can catch him, make sure you keep him hydrated. Remember to offer your child water throughout the day. This is the time to teach him to quench his thirst with water. If you constantly offer him juice he will come to expect that liquids will always have a flavor. This is not the habit you want to create.

Building Blocks of Healthy Toddlers

LET TODDLERS GRAZE Toddlers aren't going to eat three meals a day like we do. They have such little stomachs that they really do need to have food available to them throughout the day. So let toddlers graze, and remember to keep portions small.

> ▶ **TIP** Many nutritionists say that adults should eat like toddlers do: Eat when we're hungry. Stop when we're full. And eat small meals throughout the day.

HEALTHY SNACKS FOR HEALTHY KIDS When we were kids, most of our parents taught us that snacking would ruin our appetites for dinner. Today, we don't consider "no eating between meals" to be a valid rule, especially for toddlers. So why not feed them a nourishing snack when they're hungry? A healthy snack will keep them going until mealtime, keep them happy, provide the nutrients they may miss at a regular meal, and teach them to eat only till they're satisfied.

Toddlers don't equate snacks with sugar or salt. They haven't learned that yet. But what you serve your toddler now will become their snack pattern for future years, so don't provide them with unwholesome foods like sugary treats, soft drinks, imitation fruit drinks, salty chips, and pretzels. Offer your little ones nutritious snacks. Try bite-size chunks of seasonal fruits, vegetables, low-fat cheese, bits of eggs, dry cereals, whole-grain breads and muffins, a little low-fat yogurt, or a small bowl of cooked rice and milk.

Nutritionist Liz Shaio suggests cutting pieces of celery and spreading peanut butter inside the celery curve. Sprinkle raisins on top and you've got Ants on a Log! My mom had several variations on the celery snacks. She used to fill them with peanut butter, and also cream cheese and cheddar cheese. (Today, we use the low-fat versions of the cheeses.) She also kept carrot and cucumber slices in the fridge and would give them to us to hold us over to dinner. We loved them!

Another fun snack idea from Liz: Use cookie cutter shapes on low-fat cheese slices and soft fruits and vegetables, to press out stars, hearts, half moons, letters, numbers, leaves, and trees. She also suggests freezing in-season fruits, like bananas or berries, and serving them to your toddler as a frozen treat. Or whip up this delicious smoothie.

The Anytime Smoothie

½ banana

*5 strawberries

½ cup Non-Fat Yogurt (Plain)

½ cup Apple Juice

Directions:

1.   Add all ingredients into a blender and mix for 1–2 minutes.

2.   Experiment with different fruit combinations—mangoes, peaches, nectarines, blueberries, melon, pineapple, or papaya. If you want to make it a frozen treat, add ice cubes and mix at a higher speed. Tastes like a naturally sweet frozen treat.

* Make sure your toddler ate these fruits as an infant and they caused no problems. If this is the first time she's eating any of these fruits, give her the fruit first before making the smoothie to be sure she has no reaction.

WATCH THOSE HIDDEN SUGARS One thing I've discovered as I've become more health conscious is that sugar calories can mount up fast due to the many hidden sugar sources. For instance, one tablespoon of ketchup has a little over a half-teaspoon of sugar. Fruited yogurt has six teaspoons of sugar per cup! Pork and beans has almost 2½ teaspoons of sugar per half cup. Sugar is hidden in products you wouldn't even think about—like bologna.

Those of us preparing meals for our families really must use caution when buying food. It's important to take the time to read all labels carefully and to understand the information they contain. Ingredients are always listed in descending order of amount. For instance, if the label lists corn syrup as the first ingredient, it contains more sugar than any other ingredient.

Sugar by any other name is still sugar. When you're reading labels, here's what to watch out for: Corn Syrup, Corn Sweetener, Corn Sugar, Maple Syrup, Honey, Molasses, Fructose, Dextrose, Lactose, Sucrose, Glucose, Raw Sugar, Brown Sugar, and High Fructose Corn Syrup.

PUT A LID ON THE JUICE Too often, kids will fill up on juice and milk and then aren't hungry for solid foods. (Wonder why your child won't eat at mealtime?) Nutritionists advise us to limit our toddlers to 6 ounces of juice each day, and a maximum of 24 ounces of milk. The rest of their nutrients should come from food and water. Yes, water. Encourage your child to drink water when she's thirsty instead of drinking calorie-heavy beverages.

▶ TIP Nutritionist Liz Shaio says, "It's always better to eat the fruit than drink the juice—you get more fiber."

Dr. W | **Cancer-Fighting Foods**

It's not hard to follow a cancer-fighting food regime. Cut back on empty calories—high amounts of saturated fats, sugar, processed foods, and junk foods—and add fruits, vegetables, whole grains, legumes, and low-fat dairy products.

If you can't figure out how to cut back on those calories, or if you're having trouble getting your kids to eat all those cancer-fighting fruits and vegetables, the answer may be right in front of you! Look at what's on your family's dinner plates. Anytime you see fruits or vegetables in tiny, garnishlike amounts, you have an opportunity to switch ratios. Cut down on the mountains of red meat and add more of those cancer-fighting phytochemicals, antioxidants, and other substances supplied by fruits, vegetables, and whole grains.

DON'T ELIMINATE FAT Young children need fat in their diets for normal organ and cell growth, as well as brain development. Your toddler's diet should consist of no more than 30 percent fat, and no less than 20 percent fat, the same requirement for us adults.

Parents who are restricting the fat in their own diets should be careful not to impose their low-fat and non-fat foods on their little ones because fat is necessary for their developing bodies. We went to Michelle Daum, pediatric and adolescent nutritionist in Westchester, New York, who gave us the skinny on fats!

Michelle Daum

Dietary fats are essential for the health and development of your growing child. Fats provide children with a great source of energy, are necessary for growth, help prevent certain vitamin deficiencies and have other important functions. But it's vitally important for all of us to understand that not all fats are created equal. Researchers are learning that the type of fat is probably more important than the amount of fat when considering heart risk. And since we also want to avoid increasing the number of our children's fat cells and lower their risk for obesity and other chronic adult conditions, it's critical that we know which fats are helpful and which should be avoided.

SATURATED FATS: Pay particular attention to and try to limit saturated fats. They can raise levels of bad LDL cholesterol and can lead to heart disease. Saturated fats are mostly found in meat, butter, whole milk, and whole milk dairy products such as cheese, yogurt, ice cream, and cream. Vegetable oils that are saturated, coconut oil, palm oil and palm kernel oil, are found in commercial cookies, crackers, and other commercially baked products.

TRANS FATS: Trans fats, like saturated fats, raise LDL cholesterol in the blood. Trans fats are formed when a liquid fat is transformed into a solid fat. This process is called hydrogenation. Trans fats are mostly found in margarines, shortenings, crackers, cookies, cakes, cereal bars, and commercially fried foods.

To keep trans fat intake low, check the ingredient list for "hydrogenated" or "partially hydrogenated fats," choose soft margarines (liquid or tub) instead of stick margarine and limit the amount of cookies, pastries, crackers, cakes, and fast-food fries you eat.

Fortunately, the government is helping out by mandating that trans fats be listed on the Nutrition Facts panels of food labels by the year 2006.

MONOUNSATURATED FATS: These fats may help to lower blood cholesterol. But remember, monounsaturated fats are still loaded with calories. Olive oil, peanut oil, sesame seed oil, canola oil, avocados, and nuts are all high in monounsaturated fat.

POLYUNSATURATED FATS: These fats have also been shown to help reduce the risk of heart disease. Oils that are mostly polyunsaturated include: corn oil, cottonseed oil, safflower oil, sunflower oil, soybean oil, and fish oil. If weight is a concern, remember that polyunsaturated fats, like other fats, contain plenty of calories.

CULTIVATE A LOVE OF FRUITS AND VEGETABLES We've learned today that an anti-cancer diet is low-fat, high fiber, with an emphasis on fruits and vegetables. This was a message that I actually heard early on from my Dad, who was a cancer specialist and raised as a vegetarian. Naturally, he was a big proponent of vegetables in our home. He thought that if my brother, Jeff, and I helped to plant a vegetable garden, we'd probably enjoy harvesting, maybe even help cook, and most certainly have a better attitude about eating the vegetables that we planted. Boy was he right! We checked the progress of our garden daily and couldn't wait to taste the fruits (and vegetables!) of our labors. Of course, now when I read advice from parenting experts who suggest doing exactly that, I think back to my dad and realize that he was pretty smart. (Funny how that works—you only realize how smart your parents were when you become a parent yourself.)

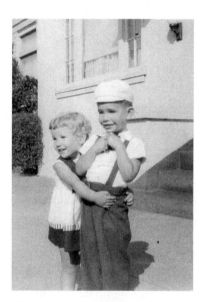

Together, we planted tomatoes, corn, zucchini, yellow summer squash, yellow crookneck squash, string beans, peas, rhubarb, and eggplant. We also planted berries, grapes, cherries, apples, kumquats, loquats, and avocado (that's when I learned that an avocado was a fruit!), and one of my dad's favorites, a quince tree.

But what I remember most is the zucchini. Boy, did we grow a lot of zucchini! My mom—Glady, as she was called—couldn't come up with enough recipes to use all the zucchini we grew. Here's one dish she served that I still make today. It's as easy as can be, and really fast and tasty.

Me at three with brother Jeff

Glady's Skillet Zucchini

1. Pour two tablespoons of olive oil into a skillet (My mom used butter, but I've become more heart healthy.)

2. Sauté half a yellow onion, sliced.

3. Add several green zucchinis sliced. I sometimes add sliced yellow squash for color.

4. Sauté a few minutes, then add 1 to 2 teaspoons of water and put a lid on the pan until the zucchini softens a little. While adults may prefer their vegetables *al dente,* young children prefer them softer. Just don't let it get too mushy.

OPTIONAL: To add another flavor and get another veggie into your meal, add sliced red bell pepper or halved cherry tomatoes to the pan. How many tomatoes you use will determine the taste. My mom has also been known to add a can of stewed tomatoes, and top the dish off with parmesan cheese.

Get Your Toddler Moving!

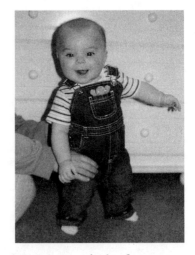

Max, striving for his first independent step.

In addition to choosing the right foods, you need the right moves to stay healthy! Exercise becomes vitally important once a child is able to walk and move. Not only does it burn up calories that are consumed, exercise also stimulates your body to produce hormones for digestion, as well as endorphins, the "feel good" hormones. And of course muscles will only develop if they are used. The toddler who is parked in front of the television rather than chasing you around is on his way to obesity.

Encouraging your children to stay active will

create the exercise habit for the rest of their lives. Consider dancing and gymnastics (little ones love to jump and tumble!), riding a tricycle, and running races in the backyard. Or what about an old-fashioned game of tag or just taking a family walk in the park? Activity and childhood go together like hugs and kisses.

Putting It All Together

Let's face it, toddlers don't know from healthy or not healthy. It's all up to us. This is our golden opportunity. Remember, young children tend to mimic behavior, so be a good role model by making wise nutritional choices and eating a variety of foods yourself. When your toddler sees you eating all those healthy foods, he'll be encouraged to enjoy fruits and vegetables, multi-grains, legumes, and milk—all of those iron-rich, calcium-rich, fiber-rich foods. Teaching your child to love healthy foods and to stay active at this young age will go a long way to ensuring a healthy life. And you can be confident that, as a parent, you are doing all you can to give your child the best chance of living disease-free.

12

Off to School

It's another rite of passage. Along with the first word, the first step, and the first fall, your child's first trip to school is bound to make you a bit misty-eyed. It's the start of an enormous adventure—a new environment with new people—for both you and your child. It's an experience that causes butterflies . . . and perhaps some tears.

Starting school is a major transition, especially for parents who've not yet experienced a previous separation. So far, your little one has been safe and secure in the loving arms of family. And up to this point, those parents whose children haven't been in childcare outside of the home have been in total control of their child's nutrition. In the past few years you've been attempting to make eating a healthy adventure. Hopefully, you've offered variety, you've cut back on high-calorie, high-fat foods, and you've introduced your child to cereals and grains, fish, an abundant array of fruits and vegetables, and some delicious healthy snacks. Perhaps you even know every morsel she's popped into her mouth. But what's going to happen now? Will your child's eating patterns change? Can you be certain she'll be eating the right foods? What can you do to insure she'll continue down the nutritionally sound path?

Be A Take-Action Parent

Now that your child is on his own (for a few hours anyway!), your job is to help her continue to make wise and healthy eating choices. It's a challenging task, but it can be made easier if you don't abdicate control. Get involved. Find out what foods the school is serving your child and, if possible, participate in your school lunch programs. Make some healthy suggestions and voice your concerns. Help your child understand how to make healthy choices even though she's away from home, and try to plan ahead so that you always have a good selection of nutritious foods on hand. If you guide your school-age child toward smart food choices now, you can help her avoid the growing obesity epidemic, and possibly protect her from a future of heart disease, Type II diabetes, high blood pressure, osteoporosis, and cancer.

> **Dr. W** *Did you know that federal regulations on the mandated caloric content of school meals date back to 1946? They were designed in response to the incidence of youth malnutrition. We've come a long way—now obesity is a far more prevalent problem among young people. But the government still demands that school breakfast programs (which serve eight million kids) provide 25 percent of the recommended dietary allowance (RDA) of calories. Further, the over twenty-eight million school lunches served daily exceed the standard for fat content and provide another third of the daily allowance. That leaves only 42 percent (less than half) of the calories recommended daily for our children's dinner and snacks.*
>
> *Serving fattening school meals may have made sense years ago, but today they should be simpler, smaller, and healthier. Why not a sliced chicken sandwich with lettuce and tomato? Who said a school lunch has to be hot?*

DO YOUR HOMEWORK Now that your child is learning her first lessons at school, this might be a good time for you to do some homework of your own and find out the best way to insure that your child receives the proper nutrients to grow up healthy. Recently, Tom Brokaw, of *NBC Nightly News,* reported the results of a new childhood obesity study from the American Academy of Pediatrics. According to Dr. John Parks of the Emory University School of Medicine, "Overweight kids become overweight adults—

and overweight adults are not only at risk for increased heart disease, but also cancer." The report goes on to say that the percentage of overweight children in the United States has doubled in the last twenty years. *More than 15 percent of 6- through 11-year-olds are now overweight.* Another study, this one from the Centers for Disease Control and Prevention, also reported that almost 20 percent of third graders and 21 percent of sixth graders in New York City are obese.

Currently, with the obesity epidemic growing larger every day, the federal government is taking a new look at the school lunchroom guidelines. In New York City, the Education Department is reducing the fat content in the 800,000 meals it serves daily and banning candy, soda, and other sugary snacks from school vending machines. School districts nationwide have been reevaluating the meals they serve and some have begun cutting back on junk food and soft drinks in cafeterias. To make sure that each meal contains no more than 30 percent fat, schools will need to use more whole wheat bread, serve more fresh fruits and vegetables, serve more fish and foods like soy-protein-based burgers and "chicken," and decrease the number of mayonnaise-based salads. Cookies and other snacks will also need to be made smaller, and beverages will need to be limited to water, milk, and juice made of 100 percent fruit.

But the fight against childhood obesity is still in its nascent phase. It's going to take a lot more work. It's time we as parents get involved and address this heartbreaking epidemic.

GET YOUR CHILDREN INVOLVED Since most school-age children want a say in what they're going to have for lunch, why not include them in the selection and preparation of their lunches. Use this time to teach them how to make healthy, tasty choices.

- Involve your children in making shopping lists.

- Make a weekly shopping date with your kids. They can help read labels, which will make them more conscious of ingredients.

- Take kids to ethnic markets—looking at all the unusual ingredients is fun and fascinating, and exposes them to the world around them.

- Listen to your child's suggestions and let them experiment with new foods.

- Encourage *them* to do some of the cooking with you.

- Experiment with new recipes together.

- Learn new culinary words—like *al dente, braise* and *marinade*.

- Ask for suggestions and let your child plan some meals.

- Explain how foods such as vegetables, fruits, milk, and whole grains help to prevent cancer, heart disease, osteoporosis, and Type II diabetes.

- Play outside together before or after dinner—run, chase, catch!

- Look for nearby parks and hiking trails where you can hike and picnic together.

PLAN AHEAD Your child's first year at school will often start a whole run of activities, from play dates, to ballet lessons, to soccer practice. And as busy as your child's life gets, yours will get even busier! That's why it's more important than ever to get organized and plan healthy meals and snacks—otherwise you might just succumb to whatever's on hand, healthy or not . . . or the closest fast-food outlet or vending machine. Stock your

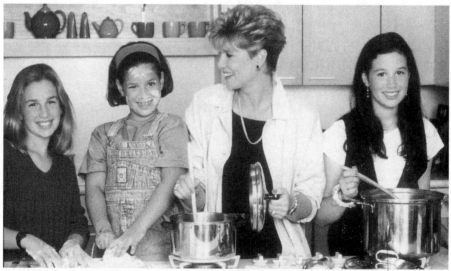

It might be messier when they help, but it's sure a lot more fun.

refrigerator and cabinets with a myriad of nutritious choices. In addition to ready-to-eat fruits and vegetables, yogurts and cheeses, also keep on hand low-salt, low-fat soups, peanut butter (natural is best with no sugar added), dried fruits, beans, whole grains, nuts, and protein energy bars. It will help you to think through the lunches you'll be preparing the next week. Be sure to include those foods on your shopping list and take it with you when you do your regular shopping.

BE FLEXIBLE Don't get hung up on what breakfast, lunch, and dinner are *supposed* to look like. It's perfectly okay to mix it up a bit. When Jamie, Lindsay, and Sarah were little they loved the idea of having what they called breakfast-dinners: veggie omelets, banana pancakes, or blueberry waffles at the traditional dinner hour. Breakfast-dinners were such a hit that the girls were always eager to pitch in. They still love to make these fun and easy meals, and wanted to share one of their favorite recipes with you.

Lindsay's Bird's Nest

1 slice whole wheat or 7-grain bread

1 egg

1 T butter

Directions:

Take a small glass (or cookie cutter), place in center of bread and cut out a circle. Place butter in pan until hot, and then place the bread in the pan. Crack an egg into the hole and cook until done. (To avoid eggshell remnants in Bird's Nest, crack the egg into a small bowl first, and then pour into the hole in the bread.)

Start the Day With a Brainpower Breakfast

When my three older daughters were young, I always tried to get them to eat in the morning before going to school. It was always a struggle! Then, one day on *Good*

Morning America, our science editor, Dr. Michael Gillen, a physics professor at Harvard University, brought a Bunsen burner onto the set. He pointed to the idle burner and said, "This is your body when you wake up in the morning." Then he lit the flame underneath the burner, and the water bubbled up. "That's breakfast," he said. "It's the energy your body needs to get going. It's what starts the engine. If you don't put any gas in your car, the engine can't start up and start burning that fuel to go forward. It's the same thing with breakfast," he continued. "If you don't put any fuel into your body in the morning, then your body can't start burning calories and move forward."

I loved that wonderful demonstration and, after the show, couldn't wait to tell my daughters who always rolled their eyes when I tried to coax them to eat breakfast with my "food is fuel for your body" theory. And of course, being a mom, I just had to add my own take. "If you don't have breakfast, then you'll be tired, you'll be lethargic, and you won't have the fuel you need to power your brain and get through the day."

You know what? I think they finally got it.

> **Dr. W** *Children who eat a balanced breakfast have higher test scores, demonstrate better behavior, are more creative, are absent less often, have more strength and energy, have lower blood cholesterol, and have less chance of becoming obese. That makes sense when you consider the essential nutrients contained in breakfast foods. For example, a glass of orange or grapefruit juice is rich in vitamin C; bread products made with whole-grain or enriched flour, or fortified breakfast cereals supply most of the needed B complex vitamins. Milk and milk products supply calcium. And nonhydrogenated margarine is usually fortified with vitamin A.*

Of course, *what* you actually eat for breakfast is also important. Breakfast should provide food selections from at least three different food groups, plus low-fat or skim milk. For example: Protein—eggs or a handful of nuts in cereal; Grains—whole-grain cereal or whole wheat toast; Fruit—melon or berries; Dairy—skim milk or low-fat yogurt. You don't want your child's breakfast to have too much fat or too much sugar. These foods will set him up for an "energy letdown" by midmorning. In fact, fat and sugar can actually make your child rather sleepy before he even gets to lunch.

My husband and I usually have a glass of orange juice in the morning. We just love it! Of course, it's even better if you serve a piece of fresh fruit. A 12-ounce glass of orange juice is derived from six large oranges, and by drinking only the fruit juice, you're getting more sugar and no natural fiber. That's not to say that there isn't a place for fruit juice at the breakfast table—juice, like the whole fruit, contains natural sugars that give your body a jump start. It's just that as take-action parents you need to know the difference.

Fruit smoothies are also nutritious breakfast choices that often contain juice *and* whole fruit. And they taste mighty darn good. My family keeps bags of frozen fruit in our freezer—strawberries, raspberries, pineapple, etc., and bananas that have been peeled and sliced so they're ready to pop into a blender.

Want some more smoothie ideas?

Joan's Breakfast Smoothie

1 cup frozen strawberries

½ orange, peeled and sectioned

½ banana, cut up (I like the bananas frozen)

⅓ cup low-fat yogurt.

Orange juice as needed.

Ice cubes will give you a frozen version!

Directions

Mix in blender. To get the right consistency, you can add a little orange juice or ice. I change the fruits all the time. I like to add raspberries and papaya; my husband likes pineapple. Mix it up and experiment—try new flavors.

Jamie-Lindsay-Sarah's Smoothie

1 frozen banana

1 cup skim milk

2 T peanut butter

Dash of vanilla

½ cup crushed ice

Directions:

Place all ingredients in the blender and mix. Delicious!

Pack a Lunch That Packs A Punch

Schools that offer pizza and French fries as alternatives to healthy meal fare are encouraging our sons and daughters to eat high-fat, nutrient-poor foods. Researchers from the University of California at San Diego recently published a study in the journal *Preventive Medicine*. They estimated that the average student consumed about 26 grams of total fat at school, 30 percent more than the 20 grams recommended, and 14 percent more saturated fat than recommended.

So what can we do? Find out what your school is serving so that you can help your child make wise choices. If possible, get involved in your school lunch program and make some healthy suggestions. Your best bet? Prepare a lunch at home, and pack it with nutrients . . . and love.

Your child's lunch should provide one-third of his daily intake of vitamins, minerals, and calories. You want to make sure that his lunch has a good source of vitamin A, B vitamins, vitamin C, and calcium. Foods rich in these nutrients also contain vitamin D, iron, protein, and carbohydrates. To prepare some kid-friendly lunches that are packed full of nutrients, just follow your ABCs!

Vitamin A: Prepare a half-cup serving of deep yellow or deep orange fruits or vegetables. Baby carrots with a favorite yogurt dip, cubed cantaloupe, peaches, nectarines, or dried apricots all supply vitamin A.

Vitamin B: Give your children some meat, low-fat cheese, peanut butter sandwiches on whole-grain bread or with whole wheat crackers. Or whip up a pasta salad with low-fat cheese and kidney beans. Consider a treat of graham crackers, oatmeal cookies with raisins, or sunflower seeds. Remember, B vitamins are found in whole grains, meats, nuts, and seeds. These foods provide B vitamins, protein, carbohydrates, and iron. For kids' lunches, pack at least two servings of grains or bread and some protein every day.

Vitamins C, D, & Calcium: Pack one half-cup of fresh strawberries, red pepper slices, or citrus fruits. Vitamin C is also found in citrus juice or in those tomatoes that you put in your child's sandwich. Low-fat dairy products, including low-fat milk or yogurt, also provide protein, vitamin D and calcium.

JOAN'S FAVORITE LUNCH BAGS Here are a few ideas my kids have loved!

This one is all about wraps—wraps of all kinds. Choose whole wheat, multigrain, sundried tomato, vegetable, or corn wraps. I fill them with a variety of shredded and chopped veggies—lettuce, sprouts, carrots, tomatoes or sundried tomatoes, cucumbers, peppers, olives—and tuna or turkey, and sometimes avocado. We also love wraps stuffed with hummus. For a change of pace, we'll use whole-wheat pita pockets instead.

Another favorite? Chef's Salad in a bag. When we prepare our dinner salad, we set aside some washed and torn

> **TIP** Keep food cool! Wrap sandwiches in plastic wrap or put in Ziploc bags. Purchase a lunch box that includes a small water bottle. Fill the bottle with water and freeze it overnight. Place in lunch box to keep food cool.
>
> If you make your child's lunch the night before, be sure you keep it in the fridge overnight. Freeze individual juice packs the night before and pack along with lunch. They'll not only keep food cool, they'll be ready to drink by lunch.

Romaine lettuce, sliced cukes, and tomatoes (or whatever veggies I'm using that night), and place them in a Ziploc bag. The next morning, I add chunks of low-fat cheese, roll up some turkey, and cut into bite-size pieces. Sometimes I place a slice of low-fat mozzarella cheese on a slice of roast beef or turkey, and roll it up. (I've been known to use both roast beef and turkey!) Cut the roll into bite-size pinwheels. I add a small packet of low-fat dressing inside the bag.

The Tuna or Salmon Nicoise Option: you can also add tuna, salmon, chickpeas, olives, half a hard-boiled egg (sliced), mandarin oranges, and feta cheese. The variety is endless!

I don't know about your kids, but mine are always hungry after school. If it's your turn to carpool for tennis or soccer, make sure to take along a nutritious treat lest they try to commandeer your vehicle to the first fast-food place they see. I remember one day when I brought out a baggy of crunchy carrots and celery sticks, another of bite-size cheese cubes, and another with broccoli florets. That's when one of the little girls in the car quipped "You know the difference between boogers and broccoli? Kids don't eat broccoli!"

For dessert, we cut in-season fresh fruit into bite-size pieces and pack in Ziploc bags. (Kids eat more fruit when it's easy to pop into their mouths.)

Prepare Nutritious Snacks

Munchies are important. Snacking is actually good for kids, and may fill in the nutrients your child might not be consuming in her regularly scheduled meals. The right mid-afternoon snack can help keep kids alert, improve memory, and enhance energy levels. The best part, a nutritious munchie can actually help to prevent your child from becoming ravenous and overeat at any meal.

Try making your own trail mix by mixing sunflower seeds, dried roasted peanuts, walnuts, raisins, dried cranberries and/or cherries, pieces of dried apricot and apple. And how about crudités for a snack? Cut up carrots, celery, broccoli, cauliflower, and those sweet, delicious grape tomatoes. My Sarah loves to snack on edamame beans—Japanese soybeans found in the fresh or frozen section of your market.

LIZ SHAIO'S AFTER-SCHOOL SNACKS Kids love snacks, so why not give them healthy, fun, and delicious treats? Here are four favorites from nutritionist Liz Shaio:

Nutty-Banana Dog

Hot dog bun

1 T peanut butter

Banana slice inside

Fun-Dipping

Baked chips or thin toast crackers

Low-fat cottage cheese (an excellent source of protein and calcium)

Mix cottage cheese with fruit, salsa, or avocado.

Veggie Potpourri

Assorted veggies cut into bite-size pieces

Guacamole, hummus, baba ghanoush (eggplant spread), or raita (cucumber/yogurt dip)

Happy dipping!

Bananas on the Run

Before you go to bed, peel a banana and sprinkle with lemon juice. Insert a Popsicle stick into the end, cover with plastic wrap, and place in freezer overnight. It's great on-the-run.

The Nutrients Your School-Age Child Needs

HOW TO USE THE FOOD PYRAMID Use the USDA Food Guide Pyramid to show you what to eat each day. It's not a rigid prescription, but a general guide that lets you choose a healthful diet that's right for you and your children.

The Pyramid shows you how to get a variety of foods that will get your child the nutrients he needs, as well as the right number of calories to maintain healthy weight.

Start with the largest group on the Food Pyramid and include 6–11 servings of whole wheat breads, cereals, rice, and pasta. Add 3–5 servings from the vegetable group, and 2–4 servings from the fruit group. Include 2–3 servings from the milk group—milk, yogurt, and cheese, and 2–3 servings from the meat group—meat, poultry, fish, dried beans, eggs, and nuts. Remember to go easy on fats, oils, and sweets, the foods in the small tip of the Pyramid. And bear in mind, portion size is important too.

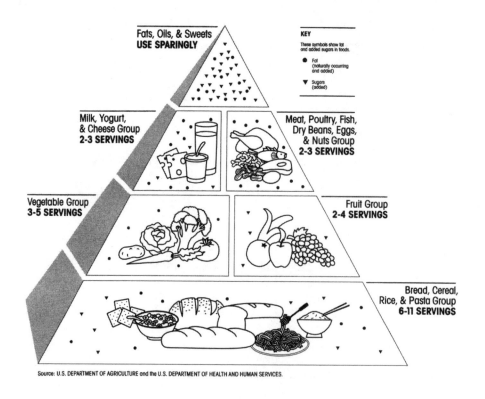

Source: U.S. DEPARTMENT OF AGRICULTURE and the U.S. DEPARTMENT OF HEALTH AND HUMAN SERVICES.

Serving Size Counts!

Listed below are portion sizes for *one serving* of each food group in the Food Pyramid.

Bread, Cereal, Rice & Pasta Group

| 1 slice of bread | = 1 ounce of ready to eat cereal | = ½ cup of cooked cereal, rice, or pasta |

Vegetable Group

| 1 cup of raw leafy vegetables | = ½ cup of other vegetables, cooked or chopped raw | = ¾ cup of vegetable juice |

Fruit Group

| 1 medium apple, banana, orange | = ½ cup of chopped, cooked, or canned fruit | = ¾ cup of fruit juice |

Milk, Yogurt, & Cheese Group

| 1 cup milk or yogurt | = 1½ ounces natural cheese, like Cheddar | = 2 ounces processed cheese, like American |

Meat, Poultry, Fish, Dry Beans, Eggs, & Nuts Group

| 2–3 ounces of cooked lean meat, poultry, or fish | = ½ cup of cooked dry beans, 1 egg, or 2 tablespoons of peanut butter |

Fats, Oils & Sweets

Use sparingly.

Dr. W Don't Forget Those Fluids

Keep your child hydrated! Water is even more essential to the body than food! A person can go for several weeks without food, but only a few days without water. Of course, your child is getting some water from fruits and vegetables, but it's not enough. Your school-aged child should be drinking eight glasses of fluids a day, more when they're active. (If your local water supply has been tested and found to be okay, tap water is fine.)

The *ABCs* of Your Child's Nutrition

When our children go off to school, we assume they'll be taught the three Rs, as they've come to be called—reading, 'riting, and 'rithmetic. However, we must never forget our responsibility to teach them the lessons of healthy living, and to help them understand that the ABCs of healthy eating go far beyond *apples, bananas,* and *carrots!* If our children are to grow into strong, healthy, disease-free adults, they must be taught what foods contain the nutrients that will offer them the protection they need. And until our school systems take this to heart, literally, it's up to us as parents to take control.

So, which foods pack a powerhouse of protection? Here are the ones that get the best grades!

BERRY GOOD! Blueberries, strawberries, raspberries, and cranberries are chock-full of vitamin C, fiber, and disease-fighting antioxidants. Throw them on breakfast cereals. Keep some in the freezer for a crunchy treat or to use in a fruit smoothie. Serve them on desserts such as berry crisps and parfaits.

BEANS, BEANS, THE MAGICAL FRUIT! We've all chanted that phrase with a chuckle, but it just so happens that beans and soy products do have a rather magical effect on our bodies. They're now well known for their cancer-fighting and cholesterol-lowering properties. Beans and soy products are packed with iron, zinc, folic acid, phytochemicals, and B vitamins. They're a wonderful source of fiber as well.

Kids love burritos and nachos, which you can layer with black beans and kidney beans. I recommend using baked tortilla chips and low-fat cheese. Another favorite at my house is Oriental stir-fry. My girls like adding tofu, a nutritious source of protein that picks up all the yummy flavors of the other healthy ingredients! My girls will also choose veggie burgers over chicken nuggets any day—they're made of soy protein and grains, and taste very much like the real thing. Other soy look-alikes include corn dogs and a ground-round substitute called "recipe crumbles." Use it in chili or burritos and your kids will never know the difference.

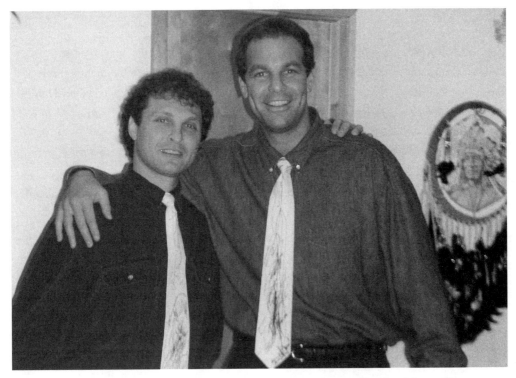

Brothers Kip and Jeff may be wearing the same tie, but only the one who drank his milk grew up to be 6'4".

SAY CHEESE—AND MILK AND YOGURT TOO This is the time when school-age children need to bank crucial stores of calcium, especially girls, who are at greater risk for osteoporosis later in life. In addition to growing strong bones, calcium may also decrease the risk of colon cancer, high blood pressure, and stroke. All children over eight should consume 1,300 milligrams of calcium a day. Again, avoid serving sodas since the phosphorous in soda is known to interfere with calcium absorption.

My best reminder of the importance of calcium comes from my husband Jeff. He always tells the story about how his older brother, Kip, hated milk. When their mom wasn't looking, Kip would always make Jeff drink his milk, too. Guess what? Today, Kip is 5 foot 10, and Jeff is 6 foot 4—ya think it was the milk?

Dr. W

Between the ages of 5 and 10, some children develop an intolerance to milk products, called lactose intolerance. Because these children lose some of the enzyme lactase, in their intestines, they are unable to break down the lactose molecules found in milk. Free lactose, or lactose that hasn't been broken down, ferments in the colon into lactic acid and produces acid stools, flatulence, and diarrhea—the symptoms of lactose intolerance. These symptoms vary with the amount of undigested lactose.

We don't know why this happens, but we do know that it affects more Asian and African-American children than Caucasian children. Although the severity of lactose intolerance varies, most children have enough lactase to digest a glass of milk in the school lunch program and small amounts of milk and milk products during the day.

COLOR YOUR WORLD Go for colorful fruits and vegetables like carrots, corn, beets, red and yellow peppers, squash, sweet potatoes, cantaloupe, and mangoes. One serving of these foods can often provide 50 to 100 percent of the daily requirement for vitamins A and C. In fact, one mango actually contains 133 percent of the daily requirement and 161 percent of the daily vitamin A requirement for children ages 4 to 6. They're really packed full of protection—fiber, potassium, and carotenoids. Mangoes and papayas make great salsas. They can add flavor to meals and replace fats.

GO FISH They don't call it brain food for nothing! Beginning with pregnancy through the second year of life, brain growth may be influenced by omega-3 fatty acids, which are plentiful in fish like salmon, tuna, and trout. Fish is also high in protein and low in fat, which is why serving it a few times a week is highly recommended.

If you fear that your picky eaters will turn up their noses at fish, start them off with something fun like fish sticks, fish burgers, or fish cakes. Make canapés for them: Spread a little light cream cheese on a cucumber slice and top it with a piece of smoked salmon, or stuff a celery stalk with white fish salad. Sometimes, getting your child to eat fish happens gradually. The mild-flavored, soft fish, like cod, halibut, or sole are good beginning fish for all children. As their taste buds develop a liking for fish, add new flavors and textures. Try shrimp, scallops, clams, or mussels mixed with pasta or rice. Experiment with my salmon burger recipe in the Recipe section.

GO WITH THE GRAIN Oatmeal, whole-grain breads, pancakes, and waffles, as well as whole-grain pasta and cereal choices provide not only fiber but also critical minerals and phytochemicals. It's important to start your kids eating high-fiber foods early on so it becomes a habit. The high-fiber habit is linked to lower cholesterol, lower risk of heart disease, lower blood pressure, and lower risk of certain cancers.

GO FOR THE GREENS Leafy greens like spinach, kale, romaine, and leaf lettuce are filled with magnesium, potassium, folic acid, carotenoids, fiber, and iron. The darker lettuces contain more vitamins than iceberg lettuce. Make interesting salads a mainstay of your meal plans, and put lettuce or spinach on your child's sandwiches.

PASS THE KETCHUP PLEASE! Here's the good news for kids who like spaghetti, and also like ketchup on their burgers. Cooked tomato products, like spaghetti sauce, tomato paste, tomato soup, and ketchup, are filled with vitamins A and C, and anti-cancer compounds such as lycopene, and other phytochemicals. However, do remember that most commercial ketchup contains sugar, so check the labels.

Be-Healthy Spelling Bee

Engage your kids in a spelling bee of a different sort. Ask them to go through the alphabet, coming up with as many healthy foods as they can for each letter of the alphabet.

As—Apples, apricots, artichokes, asparagus, and avocados.
Bs—Bananas, beets, blueberries, broccoli, and Brussels sprouts.
Cs—Cabbage, cantaloupe, carrots, cauliflower, corn, and cucumbers.

When you get to the "Ds" you can remind your child that doughnuts are just a once-in-a-while treat!

Kids Just Want To Have Fun

Why are we seeing such a trend in childhood obesity and Type II diabetes? According to the American Academy of Pediatrics the reasons for this new trend are: too much junk food, more television and video games—*and not enough exercise.* Whereas a generation ago kids may have been out playing on their own, now they're off and playing with their handheld games and watching TV. That's why parents are now advised that kids should spend fewer than two hours a day watching TV, and parents should encourage them to keep active.

Helping our children become physically active now will pay off in the long run. Children who come to expect that exercise is part of their total lifestyle are much more likely to include physical activity in their daily routines as adults. Another benefit from exercise? Typically, children who are active not only have more energy, they're better able to concentrate and excel academically.

MAKE EXERCISE A FAMILY AFFAIR Try to find some activities that you can do together as a family. I found that my girls enjoyed ice-skating, so I took to the ice . . . and have the bruises to prove it. I also wanted to make sure that we all played tennis together so

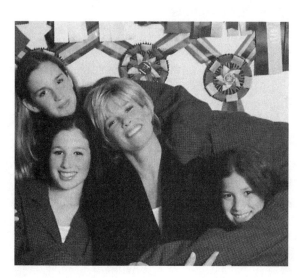

My gaggle of girls in our pjs.

they'd have that sport for the rest of their lives. That done, I got Jamie involved in horseback riding because I had enjoyed it so much as a little girl. After a few months of watching her ride around the ring and jump over the jumps with a big smile on her face, I thought, *Why did I give that up? Why don't I do that as an adult? And why don't we all do it together?* So I took up horseback riding again and soon enough, we were all going together to horse shows. For Jamie, who didn't particularly care for organized, competitive sports, horseback riding gave her an outlet where she could be physical, gain confidence, learn to persevere, and also learn responsibility for an animal. In addition, it taught her how to win and lose with dignity, and deal with disappointment. It was a great opportunity and helped shape her into the fit, competent adult she is today. Lindsay was not that keen on competitive sports either, so she turned to dance. Now an adult, she still adds jazz and hiphop to her weekly exercise routine. Sarah loves dance, too, but also played lots of Lacrosse and field hockey. My children all know that I'll never try to push them into any one particular activity—but I'll always push them to be active!

ZZZs Sleep—Getting Sleep is Just as Important as Getting Active

Deep sleep coincides with the release of growth hormone in children and young adults. During sleep, the cells of their bodies show increased production and reduced breakdown of proteins. Since proteins are the building blocks needed for cell growth and for repair of damage from factors like stress and ultraviolet rays, a good night's deep rest may truly offer children the proverbial "beauty sleep."

The National Institute of Neurological Disorders and Stroke

Not enough sleep also affects other chemicals and hormones in your child's body. Thyroid hormones, which also affect energy levels, can fluctuate. Cortisol, which helps to control levels of sugar in the blood and aids in fighting stress—whether it's the result of being chased on the playground or fighting off an infection—can be thrown off.

Sleep Center—Children's Memorial Hospital, Chicago

Putting It All Together

No longer a toddler entirely dependent on your choices, your school-age child has been developing the proverbial mind of her own, and will welcome the chance to not only participate in food and activity choices, but to be heard! What better time to teach your children to make smart food choices that will fuel their brain power and their bodies? As parents, we offer them the first line of protection against becoming part of the obesity epidemic, and their best chance at avoiding a future of heart disease, Type II diabetes, high blood pressure, osteoporosis, and cancer.

Take this opportunity to make healthy living a family affair . . . and to make it fun! Don't pressure your child to eat. If you battle over food, you will lose. And don't overly focus on the details of what they are eating. Involve your child in the selection and preparation of wholesome meals and snacks. Be a good role model. Your children learn from you, so set the right example. Eat a nutritious dinner together as a family whenever possible, and find activities to do together. Go on family hikes, run in the park, play tennis, soccer, and baseball. Rent a kayak, buy some weights and lift them together, or adopt a dog and let your kids be in charge of walking her. Limit your child's time on the Internet and in front of the TV. In fact, everyone in the family should get up from the couch and out from behind the computer and get involved with each other. That way you can all be healthy together.

13

Adolescence—
Life in the Fast-Food Lane

Your teenager looks at you as if *you* were born yesterday; the telephone rings and it's never for you. Your son worries about acne. Your daughter turns up with strange piercings in places other than her ears. Their rooms are a mess—dirty clothes are strewn all over the floor. And just how many burgers, fries, and sodas can they consume?

Adolescence is a time of rapid physical development and deep emotional change. Your teenager's body is now producing hormones. Your daughter begins menstruating; your son's voice cracks and lowers. And don't forget that sudden fragility and moodiness. This period between childhood and adulthood can be a minefield for parents and adolescents alike. You want to let your kids test their independence, but you also want to make sure that they stay safe, and of course healthy. As parents, you want to make sure that your children continue to eat nutritious foods and keep up with the healthy habits they've learned in their early years, but so much seems to be out of your control now you wonder if that's even possible. So, what can you do to help your teenager navigate life in the fast-food lane?

Be a Take-Action Parent

We're blessed that many of our teenaged sons and daughters have taken the anti-smoking message to heart, but what about good nutrition and the perils of obesity? Despite an abundance of available material on the subject, it seems like most of our teenagers don't really understand the consequences of a poor diet or inactive lifestyle, and still don't regard the obesity message as serious. They're not aware that along with the emotional stings of being overweight, obesity is also a risk factor for many adult diseases—Type II diabetes, heart attacks, stroke, cancer, and high blood pressure. But the statistics are truly startling: since 1975, adolescent obesity rates have tripled! So while our teenagers have been making their strikes for independence, they've gotten fatter. As take-action parents it's up to us to help them pay attention to what they're eating and to get them to realize the value of good, nutritious foods.

BEWARE OF SUPER-SIZED KIDS Our adolescents are shoveling more and more super-sized fast foods into their mouths: burgers, tacos, pizza-with-extra-cheese, fried chicken, hoagies, double fries, ice cream, and doughnuts. Although fast-food restaurants have been around for a long time, in the past two decades, portion sizes have increased. Fast-food fare advertises and serves giant sodas, super-sized burgers, jumbo tubs of popcorn, extra cheese, double meat, colossal muffins, and king-sized fries. In 1977, the average hamburger weighed 5.7 ounces. In 1996, it grew to 7 ounces, which is nearly 100 extra calories. Soft drinks also went from 12 ounces to almost 20 ounces—another 100-calorie increase. And the portions continue to grow ever larger.

Writing in the *New York Times,* health and science columnist Erica Goode reports that "portion size, price, advertising, the availability of food and the number of food choices presented—can influence the amount the average person consumes." And that includes our teenagers, who are gobbling up these mammoth servings and becoming the tribe of the overweight. Low-cost fast food has lured a lot of our teenagers into a high-fat trap. If your teenager frequents a fast-food joint three times a week—or more!—suggest he cut back to once a week for a while, and then to twice a month. Small changes in a teenager's eating pattern can equal a large payoff over time.

Dr. W

Not too long ago, fourteen-year-old Brandon, the overweight son of a friend, pleaded with his parents to go to a particular restaurant. "They give you double cheese, double meat, and double fries," he explained. When his mother expressed concern, Brandon added, "Don't worry, Mom, it's all for under four dollars!"

Like Brandon, many teenagers believe that getting a lot for their money is something that will make their parents proud. They don't correlate eating fat-laden fast foods with the risk of disease later in life. It happens in almost every family. Peer pressure begins to erode a lot of the sound nutritional direction you thought you had instilled in your child.

Be Aware of Portion Distortion

As portion sizes get larger . . . so do our kids. A recent study by the Centers for Disease Control and Prevention examined American's eating habits for the past 30 years. They concluded that the rising rate of obesity is due in part to oversized portions. The researchers found that during this 30-year period (1971–2000), serving sizes became 2–5 times larger. I think a lot of us have lost track of what a portion is supposed to be. So, what does three ounces of cooked meat look like? How big are two teaspoonfuls of peanut butter? Here's a handy reference guide to help you to understand what an appropriate portion *really* looks like.

½ cup of fruit, vegetables, cereal, pasta, or rice equals a small fist.

3 ounces of cooked meat equals a deck of cards.

1 muffin equals a large egg.

1 teaspoon of butter equals one thumb tip.

2 tablespoons of peanut butter equals a golf ball.

A small baked potato equals the size of a computer mouse.

1 ounce of cheese equals two dice.

4 small cookies equal four casino chips.

A pancake or waffle equals a 4-inch CD.

From the International Food Information Council.

WATCH OUT FOR FAST FOOD AT SCHOOL Super-sizing isn't the only overweight land mine teenagers are stepping onto. Did you know that among adolescents the most popular lunchtime foods are subs, burgers, and pizza? Since easy access to fast foods makes it more likely that your adolescent's diet will be higher in fat and calories and lower in fruits and vegetables, why are fast foods so readily available in our schools? Because before we started paying attention, fast-food companies began targeting children through TV ads, games, and contests. They then crossed the last advertising and sponsorship frontier to enter school cafeterias and school lunch programs. For schools dealing with major budget slashing, fast-food revenue looked like an answer. No one counted on creating a new population of overweight kids.

In response to the growing obesity epidemic, some cities and states are taking steps to reverse the fast-food trend in their school food programs. California's Project LEAN, administered by the Public Health Institute, was created to look at the impact that the à la carte fast-food program has on the current and future eating habits of teenagers. Project LEAN is implementing programs that promote the link between a nutritious diet and learning. Their mission is to offer students more healthy foods that are just as convenient, inexpensive, and appealing as fast foods. To accomplish this goal, administrators are using taste tests, surveys, and classroom discussions to involve students in choosing healthy foods for their school. (For more information on Project LEAN, go to: www.californiaprojectlean.org.)

GET TEENS BACK ON THE PLAYING FIELD School budget slashing has not only taken its toll on school lunch programs, but physical fitness programs have also felt the monetary crunch. And many have even been eliminated! Our teenagers aren't exercising enough, which is also fueling the obesity epidemic. Reporting on the exercise crisis, here's what the Centers for Disease Control and Prevention tells us:

- Nearly half of American youths aged 12–21 years old are not vigorously active on a regular basis.

- About 14 percent of young people report no recent physical activity.

- Participation in all types of physical activity declines *strikingly* as age or grade in school increases.

- Only 19 percent of all high school students are physically active for 20 minutes or more, 5 days a week, in physical education classes.

Compounding the exercise problem, many parents are noticing that their teenagers are rarely outside playing ball on weekends or after school. The only sports they seem to be interested in are surfing the Web, Instant Messaging, downloading music, playing video games, and chatting on the phone. Inactivity is adding to our adolescents' weight problems. To prevent them from becoming fatter and less healthy, we need to get them moving.

KNOW THAT YOUR KIDS ARE WATCHING YOU Is there anyone left who hasn't downed a pint of ice cream when life's been a little rough and disappointing? Whether it's fudge ripple, a package of chocolate-chip cookies, fried chicken and mashed potatoes, or a large bag of barbecue-flavored potato chips that sings to you, by calling these choices "comfort foods," we're giving them extraordinary power. When our kids watch us gobble down and slurp up these foods after a bad day, they're learning that food is a source of emotional comfort, and they will mimic our behavior. While there are no good foods or bad foods, by showing our kids that *any* food has the power to console, we could be setting them up for a lifetime of weight problems, with all of the attendant risks.

PREPARE FOR PANTRY RAIDS Although you're never going to be able to control your teenager's forays into fast-food eating when she's out of the house, you still can exert some control over what she puts into her belly while she's under your roof. I've found that by stocking my cabinets, freezer, and refrigerator with bite-size ready-to-eat nutritious foods, my family was better able to make the transition from sodium-filled, fat-laden, sugar-loaded junk food to a wide variety of healthful, tasteful treats.

- My freezer is loaded with frozen strawberries, raspberries, grapes, bananas (for smoothies anytime), edamame (fresh frozen soybeans), whole-grain waffles, veggie burgers, fresh fruit pops, and low-fat frozen yogurt bars.

- My refrigerator is stocked with: sliced raw veggies—lettuce, cucumbers, baby carrots, celery, and cherry tomatoes, all in small containers; cut-up fruit—melon, peaches, apples, watermelon, pineapple, nectarines, strawberries, and apricots; slices of low-fat turkey and chicken; chunks of low-fat cheese; whole wheat pita and tortillas for wraps; tubs of low-fat salsa, low-fat sour cream, fat-free yogurt, hummus, low-fat mayo, and low-fat cream cheese; skim milk, homemade lemonade, natural fruit juices, and lots and lots and lots of bottled water.

- The cabinets in my kitchen are stocked with cans of chickpeas, tuna fish in water, salmon, kidney beans, black beans, and red beans. I also keep individual cups of vegetarian soups, rice cakes, raisins, low-fat protein bars, popcorn (but not with butter and salt), baked tortilla chips, fortified cereals (be sure to check the label for hidden sugar!), low-fat granola, low-fat/low-sugar cookies, peanut butter, almond butter, tahini, almonds, walnuts, sugarless jams and jellies, and dried fruit.

As you can see, my kitchen is brimming with great things to eat that my kids have learned to love! It took some time for all of us to get used to a new way of healthy eating, but by keeping the selections interesting, tasty, and *available,* we eventually began to crave these foods instead of our old fat-and-sugar-laden fare.

Dr. W *Although most adolescents eat three meals a day, they get only about 80 percent of their calories at mealtime—the other 20 percent comes from snacks. Breaking up the total food intake into a number of smaller meals is actually more healthy than limiting food intake to three meals a day, as long as the snacks are healthy. Your snacking adolescent may have replaced the standard eating pattern with a much better one. By snacking, he's avoiding the large-portion, stuffed-belly syndrome.*

GET YOUR TEENAGER INVOLVED IN MEALTIME Try to get your adolescents involved in grocery shopping and cooking! Ask them to help prepare the shopping list, go to the grocery store with you, and, while you're there, read the food labels together.

Allow your teens to experiment in the kitchen, and be sure to let them know how much you appreciate their creations. Teenagers who make their own food decisions are more likely to make healthy choices.

GET READY FOR GROWTH SPURTS Children usually grow at a gradual, steady pace until they reach puberty, when they experience an intense spurt in growth. In fact, the last time they grew this quickly was in infancy (when they were much easier to control!).

Girls experience their growth spurt around the age of 10 or 11, usually preceding their entry into puberty, and peak by age 12. At the end of the spurt, they'll have grown approximately 3½ inches taller and gained about 20 pounds.

Boys don't start their growth spurts until age 12 to 13, and reach their peak at 14. During the growth spurt, boys add about 4 inches in height and gain about 23 pounds.

But adolescents aren't just getting taller and heavier. As they mature into young adults their body shape is changing along with their height and weight. Soon after the spurt in height begins, muscle growth increases rapidly. Their bodies are changing so swiftly that they often experience what's commonly called "growing pains."

The two surest signs that adolescents are undergoing a growth spurt are: (1) their shoes and clothes become too small, and (2) there's never any food left in the fridge.

Dr. W *Your adolescent's growth spurt may allow your child to grow out of what looks like obesity. Often, normal growth during adolescence is your child's strongest weight-regulating ally. Watch out for diets—they can interfere with normal growth and can be self-defeating, especially unbalanced fad diets. Low-carbohydrate, high-fat diets are low in many essential nutrients, including most of the water-soluble vitamins, complex carbohydrates (the main source of B vitamins), and other nutrients. High-carbohydrate diets are low in protein, iron, and zinc, as well as some of the fat-soluble vitamins. The only safe diet is a balanced one. This means eating a varied diet, but eating less.*

Nutrients Your Adolescent Needs

Between growth spurts, fast foods, and inactivity, your adolescent needs a lot of nutrients—vitamins and minerals, protein, complex carbohydrates, and calories. Adolescent boys need 3,000 calories a day; adolescent girls require 2,400. But along with understanding how many calories they need, it's equally important to know which foods are supplying those calories. Teenagers rarely eat the varied diet necessary to supply the important nutrients they need to support their growth and future health.

So, what nutrients do they need?

THE VITAMINS During adolescence, the requirements for virtually all vitamins increase. Teenagers should be getting their vitamins from their meals, but as you can see, that's probably not happening. Their diets are usually in short supply of essential nutrients, and as they grow older they are at risk for certain deficiencies that could lead to adult diseases.

The vitamins typically in short supply in the teenager's fast-food diet are folic acid and vitamins A and C. To ensure an adequate supply of vitamins, use the selections below as a guide.

Vitamin A: An antioxidant, it aids vision and is essential for immune system defense. This vitamin helps to form and maintain skin and mucous membranes.

Sources of Vitamin A: asparagus, blackberries, broccoli, cabbage, cantaloupe, carrots, chard, cherries, collard greens, escarole, grapefruit, kale, lettuce, mangoes, nectarines, onions (green), pears, peas, peppers (green, red, and yellow), plums, pumpkin, raspberries, squash, sweet potatoes, tomatoes, watercress, and watermelon.

Vitamin C: Also called ascorbic acid, vitamin C has many functions. As an antioxidant, it aids in bone, teeth, and gum growth, and enhances iron absorption and wound healing. It's also important in the formation of collagen.

Sources of Vitamin C: broccoli, cabbage, cantaloupe, cauliflower, grapefruit, honeydew, oranges, orange juice, potatoes, strawberries, and tomatoes.

Folic Acid: Aids in protein metabolism and promotes red blood cell formation.

Sources of Folic Acid and other B Vitamins: beans, bread (seven grain), black-eyed peas, bulgur (cracked wheat), cabbage, cereals (fortified), endive, graham flour, lettuce, limes, mangoes, oatmeal, papaya, peanuts, pearl barley, spinach, strawberries, tangerines, whole-grain corn, whole rye, and whole wheat.

THE MINERALS Like vitamins, your adolescent needs an increase in three essential minerals: calcium, zinc, and iron.

Calcium: Your teenager needs more calcium now than at any other time in her life! About 45 percent of her bones are being formed, and calcium absorption is at a high. And here's where you, as a parent, must come in to make sure that your teenager is getting sufficient amounts of low-fat dairy products and avoiding too much phosphorus-laden soda.

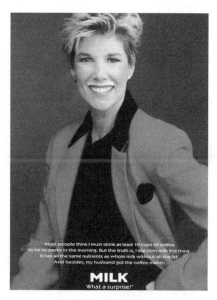

Writing in his book *Fast Food Nation,* author Eric Schlosser tells us, "In 1978, the typical teenage boy in the United States drank about seven ounces of soda every day; today he drinks nearly three times that amount, deriving 9 percent of his daily caloric intake from soft drinks. Soda consumption among teenaged girls has doubled within the same period, reaching an average of twelve ounces a day."

If your teenager is a big fan of sodas, now is the time to make some important changes. Phos-

This campaign made drinking milk cool.

phorus-laden sodas inhibit calcium absorption, disrupt good bone growth, and could be setting your teenager up for osteoporosis later in life.

Some teenagers rebel against drinking milk, so you can offer some of these other low-fat, calcium-rich foods.

Sources of Calcium: Broccoli, cereals (with milk), cheese, chocolate pudding (made with milk), cottage cheese, yogurt, custard, ricotta cheese, salmon, sardines (canned), soups (milk-based), and tofu (processed with calcium). Also look for calcium fortified foods such as juices, cereals, and other bread products.

Zinc and Iron: Zinc requirements are less clearly established than those for calcium. Zinc is necessary for growth, healing, and the formation of protein. Iron aids energy and strengthens the blood supply. An overt zinc deficiency is particularly serious in adolescents. Since zinc and iron deficiencies are closely linked, choosing iron-rich foods will provide your teenager with his necessary zinc requirement.

Sources of Zinc and Iron: Apricots (dried), beans (dried), beef, breads and cereals (iron- and zinc-fortified), greens, lamb, lentils, liver, molasses, oysters, peas (dried), prunes, sardines, spinach, tofu, and turkey.

Dr. W *When an adolescent girl begins to menstruate regularly, she's at risk for developing an iron deficiency. Ask her physician to check her iron levels regularly. If she develops an iron deficiency, be sure she takes a daily iron supplement. (Of course, even before she starts to menstruate, she should be eating a diet rich in iron to build up her reserves.)*

An adolescent boy rarely becomes iron deficient. However, after his growth spurt, particularly if he's grown a lot, his blood volume increases greatly, and he, too, should be tested for an iron deficiency. If he's deficient, he should be given an iron supplement, but only until the deficiency disappears. At that point—stop! Since high iron stores may be a risk factor for heart attacks later in life, we don't want to store too much iron in boys.

Protein: Your teenager's requirement for protein will also increase, more for boys than girls. The demands made by boys' bodies are greater—they're growing more muscle tissue. Protein supplies energy, helps build and repair tissues, forms enzymes, hormones, and antibodies to fight infections.

Sources of Protein: Low-fat dairy products, eggs, fish, lean meats, and peanut butter. Combinations like rice and beans or peanut butter on whole wheat bread also supply adequate amounts of good-quality protein.

Dr. W *Watch those saturated fats and trans fats in your teenager's diet! Although you don't want to restrict any foods, let him eat fat sparingly. Cutting back will help him to avoid the risk of heart disease, stroke, high blood pressure, Type II diabetes, and cancer.*

The Care and Feeding of Your Adolescent

YOUR TEENAGED ATHLETE Whether your teenaged athlete is a tennis player, a swimmer, a skater, a gymnast, a ball player, or an equestrian, nothing is more important to her ability to perform than good nutrition and proper hydration. Eating the right foods will help her to maintain desirable body weight, stay physically fit, and establish optimum nerve-muscle reflexes.

During rigorous training, competition, or a big game, energy requirements can reach 6,000 calories a day. If you have a teenaged athlete at home, you need no reminder—your food costs will tell you all you need to know!

Young athletes must adjust their energy intake to their output of physical activity. But getting your teenaged athlete to fuel-up properly is not always as easy as it sounds. My daughter Jamie started jumping horses competitively at age eight and developed into a national equestrian champion. But getting her to eat the proper foods and drink enough water before and during competitions was always a struggle. As she entered adolescence (and of course didn't need my advice anymore) it became even more diffi-cult. However, when she had a disappointing day or was injured, she would usually concede that it happened because she didn't have enough energy. Teenagers can be pretty smart in hindsight.

AN EATING GAME PLAN Eating the right foods is as important to your teenaged athlete's performance as expert coaching. And there's an added benefit: your adolescent's desire to improve his game offers you, as a parent, an excellent opportunity to establish sound eating practices for your entire family.

Your teenaged athlete is burning up more calories than you can imagine! To keep her endurance and strength maximized, she'll need a balanced diet with a wide variety of foods.

Starting the day with a good solid breakfast is imperative. Give her a delicious, nutrient-packed breakfast burrito and a piece of fruit, or oatmeal with fruit, or whole wheat toast with peanut butter and slices of melon. And don't forget the low-fat milk! If your young athlete hates breakfast, suggest a shake made with protein powder, fruit, and milk, or a yogurt fruit smoothie. You might want to slip a protein bar into her back-pack on her way out the door!

Lunch, dinner, and snacks should provide as much nutritious food as your athlete wants to eat, but again, include a wide variety. Many teen athletes will want to eat more servings than recommended. For instance, your 160-pound running back could gobble up as many as eight servings of bread and cereals, five servings of vegetables and fruit, and three servings of meat. Let's face it, large male teen athletes will want to eat more than the upper end of the recommended serving levels—and that's just fine.

CARB LOADING The night before the New York City marathon, all participants are invited to carb-loading pasta dinners at Tavern on the Green. In fact, every major marathon city does the same. There's good reason for these prerun events: Carb-loading increases glycogen levels in muscles and improves endurance and performance.

Complex carbohydrates should make up the bulk of the 3,000 to 5,000 calories adolescent athletes need on a daily basis. These carbohydrates will supply the extra vita-mins and minerals needed. But don't forget the protein! Your young athlete should also be eating lean meats, turkey, chicken, fish, and low-fat dairy products—skim milk, hard cheeses, and low-fat yogurt. Good nutrition is essential to any successful athletic training program.

Dr. W *Studies have shown that glycogen stores can be raised, particularly in muscle tissue, by first removing and then reintroducing dietary carbohydrates. Six days before an athletic competition, your adolescent should eat only protein and fats, and drink a lot of fluids. Three days before the competition, reintroduce only carbohydrates, and load, load, load!*

Your Teenaged Vegetarian

Don't be surprised if your adolescent comes home one night and announces: "From now on, I'm not eating meat!" I remember when my daughter Jamie made this claim. She also added, "It's cruel to animals" (she still loves all animals). Of course, once she made the decision she didn't have a clue as to what her new vegan diet should contain. Don't despair and try not to be discouraging. No matter what kind of vegetarian he or she wants to become, a well-managed vegetarian diet will meet your adolescent's nutritional needs.

Your first task is to find out the kind of vegetarian diet your adolescent intends to follow, so that you'll be able to help her replace any missing nutrients in her meals. Vegetarian regimens vary—some are more restrictive than others. Here are five vegetarian diet options:

- *Semivegetarian:* no red meat but includes some dairy products, eggs, poultry, and seafood.

- *Lacto-ovo-vegetarian:* no meat, poultry, or seafood, but includes milk, milk products, and eggs.

- *Lacto-vegetarian:* no meat, poultry, seafood, or eggs, but includes milk and milk products.

- *Ovo-vegetarian:* no meat, poultry, seafood, or milk, but includes eggs.

- *Vegan:* no animal products of any kind, including gelatin and honey.

WHAT YOUR TEENAGE VEGETARIAN NEEDS

Calcium, Dairy Products, and Saturated Fat! Much like any other diet, vegetarian diets contain a few pitfalls that need to be addressed. Most vegetarian diets have the potential of being low in calcium. If your adolescent is eating eggs, milk, cheese, poultry, or seafood, all of her calcium requirements will be met. But here's the caveat: dairy products and eggs are high in saturated fats. Use substitutions—low-fat dairy products or rice milk instead of full fat; egg white omelets a few times a week instead of whole eggs; olive oil and non-trans-fat margarine for butter.

Dark leafy vegetables, beans, and fortified orange juice also will help your adolescent protect her bones from osteoporosis and avoid the risk of developing high cholesterol, which can lead to heart disease.

Potential B$_{12}$ Deficiencies A strict vegetarian diet may be deficient in vitamin B$_{12}$, which is only provided by animal products. Since vitamin B$_{12}$ is important for producing new red blood cells, by restricting this vitamin your teenager may be at risk for anemia.

Since symptoms of this deficiency can take years to develop and are often overlooked until the late stages, it's extremely important for your adolescent vegetarian to include vitamin B$_{12}$ foritifed foods or B$_{12}$ supplements to avoid this deficiency.

Dr. W | *Iron is essential for your vegetarian teenagers. They'll need to include a lot of whole grains, beans, nuts, and dark green leafy vegetables, along with foods rich in vitamin C to insure that the iron will be absorbed properly. For example: top your young vegetarian's cereal with strawberries, or serve veggie burgers topped with tomatoes.*

Adolescent Eating Disorders

As parents, we're flooded with information about the teenagers down the street who became anorexic or bulimic. We wonder if we're doing the best possible job to protect our children from eating disorders, and if we even know the signs. Because this is such a significant adolescent problem, we asked Dr. Diane Mickley, an eating disorder expert, and founder and director of The Wilkins Center in Greenwich, Connecticut, to give us an update on this serious adolescent problem.

Dr. Diane Mickley

Sadly, even as the average weight of the American population grows heavier, our culture still equates thinness with success and happiness, even though only about 2 percent of the population has the ultrathin supermodel body type. In spite of that statistic, most normal-weight women see themselves as too heavy.

Body dissatisfaction and dieting have become the norm even among elementary school children. A recent study in New York showed that 50 percent of girls develop disordered eating sometime during their teens. About 1 percent of suburban teenaged girls develop anorexia nervosa (significant weight loss and cessation of periods), and about 5 percent of college women develop bulimia (binging and purging).

Eating disorders aren't caused by a single factor but rather the intersection of several. First off, some teenagers clearly inherit a susceptibility to eating disorders. Anorexia or bulimia occur more commonly in families with mood disorders (like depression), anxiety disorders, or alcoholism, and the latest research is beginning to identify the genes that are responsible. Secondly, certain temperaments are especially vulnerable to eating disorders. An anorexic child may be a perfectionist, sensitive, accomplished, responsible, and restrained. In contrast, the youngster who becomes bulimic may be moody and impulsive.

The developmental demands of adolescence are the key catalysts for eating disorders. Anorexia commonly occurs around age 12, right around puberty. At that age, girls become both bigger and fatter—their body fat increases from 18 percent up to 24 percent. Growth spurts cause a major increase in weight as well as in height. Boys' bodies become leaner during puberty, falling from 18 percent to 15 percent body fat.

In addition to the physical changes of the teens, there are enormous psychological demands. The approach of separation, especially for children with close families, contributes to a second peak of anorexia around 17 years of age. Bulimia typically begins later, sometimes during high school (or occasionally middle school) but onset peaks in the college years. During this time, teens are negotiating the challenges of greater independence, peer pressure, and dating. It's not too difficult to understand why teenagers would be under the misconception that losing a few pounds will make these challenges easier, and perhaps drive a vulnerable youngster to extremes.

Obesity is one of our major public health issues, and yet, so many teenagers diet to excess. Eating disorders are all too common and extremely dangerous. Ironically, some of our best and brightest young people—the most gifted and accomplished students and athletes—have a predisposition for eating disorders. Anorexia nervosa has the highest mortality of any psychiatric disorder. It is associated with heart problems, the rapid development of osteoporosis, and impaired fertility. At our center, some of the bulimic women who delay treatment until their thirties have already lost all their teeth. The psychological toll is equally devastating. Eating disorders can undermine confidence and development, and give rise to depression and a plaguing preoccupation with food. Sufferers become isolated and their relationships damaged. Because of the misery inflicted by these illnesses, even suicide can result.

The Symptoms

Weight Loss: Concerned parents should be aware of anorexia's three cardinal symptoms. The first is weight loss, to be more specific, 15 percent below ideal body weight. For a girl whose normal weight is 130 pounds, that would mean a drop in weight to 110. Preteens may grow taller, but not catch up in terms of weight. For example, let's say you have a daughter who is 75 pounds, and four feet nine inches tall. If, when she reaches five feet one inch, she only weighs 80 pounds, she has a problem.

Distorted Body Image: The second cardinal symptom is a distorted body image—your daughter continues to feel fat even though she's actually underweight. Many anorexic youngsters listen as their family or friends tell them that they're too thin, but they still see themselves as overweight, or as having a fat stomach or heavy thighs. Other anorexics may acknowledge the need for weight gain, but are unable to eat more food. Although dangerously thin, anorexics fear fatness. They believe that just going from 91 pounds to 92 will unleash an inexorable process leading to obesity.

Absence of Periods: Finally, the third cardinal symptom for girls is the absence of periods. This can occur even before any weight is lost and may be incorrectly attributed to her increased exercise. Younger girls may have developed signs of puberty, like underarm hair, but their periods don't arrive as expected even after another two years. (Girls taking birth control pills will not experience this symptom.) Interestingly, boys who become anorexic also lose hormones and develop very low testosterone levels.

Other clues you may want to watch for include increased exercise, a preoccupation with food and weight, sadness or irritability, and evasiveness or anger at the mention of restrictive eating.

About half of all anorexics are also bulimic. Most children with bulimia are in the normal weight range, though some have a history of being overweight. Bulimics share with anorexics an overvaluation of thinness—they view it as a guarantee of greater popularity, better relationships, more confidence, and happiness.

Bulimics binge—they eat excessively, feel out of control, uncomfortable, and then guilty. A binge may consist of a large volume of food (a whole pizza or cake or gallon of ice cream), but it can also be perceptual (a normal family meal that exceeds the self-restricting limit of 400 calories a day). Because of their intense longing for thinness, bulimics are driven to compensate for the calories they consume during a binge by fasting, extreme periods of exercise, or by purging. Most bulimics induce vomiting, while others may abuse diet pills, water pills, or laxatives in the mistaken notion that this will make them thinner.

In addition to youngsters with classic anorexia or bulimia, an even greater number of teens experience mild or partial versions. While they may not be 15 percent underweight or aren't purging frequently, they usually have a distorted body image and may have no menstrual periods. These teens present a wonderful opportunity for early intervention. Without treatment, however, within a few years, almost half of them will go on to a full-blown eating disorder.

The good news for young people with eating disorders is that the majority can achieve a complete cure, especially if they receive specialized, comprehensive, state-of-the-art treatment. The earlier parents recognize the symptoms and intervene, the better the outcome. Providing thorough and intensive treatment reduces the likelihood for relapse and heightens the chance for complete and permanent recovery.

Modern treatment typically uses an experienced eating disorder team— medical, nutritional, psychological, and pharmacological—to treat the teen. Full recovery often involves more than a resolution of the eating disorder symptoms. It seeks to help the teen improve self-esteem and develop better coping skills, which sets them up for an overall healthier transition to adulthood.

Dr. Diane Mickley is the founder and director of the Wilkins Center in Greenwich, Connecticut. An internist who specializes in eating disorders and weight control, Dr. Mickley has treated over 3,500 patients with these problems over the past twenty years.

Dr. W

A team approach to eating disorders is an excellent way to treat your teenager. But no matter which approach you choose—and I cannot stress this too strongly—while in recovery, vitamin and mineral supplementation is mandatory.

Vitamin deficiencies, particularly the B vitamins, rarely show themselves when the body is in a starved state. The main job of many B vitamins is to help burn calories. The fewer the calories consumed, the smaller the quantities of certain B vitamins necessary. But during rehabilitation, as your teenager's calorie intake increases, unless she is supplemented with adequate amounts of vitamins, a full-blown vitamin-deficiency disease may occur.

Discuss supplementation with your teenager's physician.

Putting It All Together

As a parent, you may feel that it's way too late to change *anything* about your adolescent, especially her eating habits. Of course, influencing your child's eating preferences is easier before they reach puberty, but I believe that as long as your kids are living at home, you still have an opportunity to effectively provide them with good nutritional guidance.

Yes, it may seem like the odds are stacked against you. Teenagers love doing things on their own terms, and they sure love hanging out at those fast food places. In fact, a recent study by Children's Hospital in Boston found that nearly one third of American kids aged 4 to 19 eat fast food daily, adding six extra pounds per year! Teenage obesity rates have more than tripled in the past twenty years. If trends like these persist, obesity will soon become the nation's number one preventable killer—overtaking smoking!

While U.S. congress says that we can't lay all the blame on the fast food industry, we have seen McDonald's step up to the plate and agree to stop supersizing their meals. It sure is a good place to start.

But what does that mean for us as parents? Perseverance and patience! You may even have to alter your own eating and exercise habits to become a good role model for them. But think about the idea that the food and activity changes you institute at this time in their lives could make the difference between a future of chronic, debilitating disease and a future of robust good health lasting well into their nineties.

PART III

The Tools

14

Your Family Medical Diary— a Gift Your Child *Cannot* Do Without!

Of all the gifts we give our children, the one they cannot do without is the gift of knowledge that is their family's medical history. We now know that there is a link between childhood nutrition and adult disease, and we also know that it is in childhood that steps need to be taken to effectively diagnose, treat, and possibly prevent chronic illnesses. Obesity, heart attack, stroke, heart disease, high blood pressure, Type II diabetes, cancer, and osteoporosis reveal themselves later, in adult years, sometimes even the late adult years. And all of these diseases have multiple causes acting simultaneously—an interaction between genetics and the environment.

We can control some important environmental factors—nutrition and exercise— to lower the risk of these diseases. But let's not forget the genetic component. Although we can't alter our genes, we can find out if our children are genetically prone to any one of these diseases and put maximum effort into helping them develop the patterns that will lower their risk for that disease. So, how do we go about obtaining this genetic information?

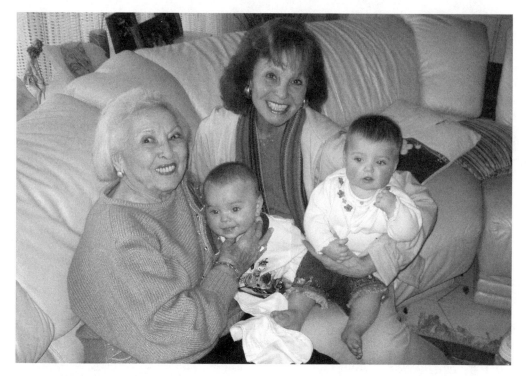

Passing family history from oldest to youngest. Great-grandma Rosie at 94, with Grandma Janey and the twins.

The Telling and the Testing— Your Family Health Diary

The best way to gather genetic information is through a carefully researched family medical history. If you are a parent or if you're preparing to become a parent, start collecting as much health data on your family as possible. Call it your Family Health Diary and update it as often as possible. We've included sample pages to insure your Family Health Diary is as complete as possible.

THE TELLING Begin by seeking out the oldest living members of the family, probably grandparents, but maybe even great-grandparents. Since the questions you'll be asking are personal and sensitive, explain that you need this information to help your pediatrician or family physician make certain decisions about treating their grandchild or great-grandchild. Then talk to any first-degree relatives of the family member you are interviewing—their brothers or sisters. If you can't talk to them directly, ask others in the family about their medical history. And be sure to ask your own parents about their history and yours.

Write all of this information in a diary, your Family Health Diary. It will be of great use not only in helping your child today but also someday in the future, when it will be useful in helping your grandchildren and great-grandchildren.

Find out what caused the deaths of their parents or grandparents, if anyone had any of the diseases we're discussing. For example, were their parents or grandparents overweight? Were they obese? Did anyone have high blood pressure? Did anyone survive cancer? Did anyone fracture a hip or other bones in old age? Did anyone have a heart attack or stroke? How about diabetes? And be sure to ask the family member you're interviewing whether he or she has had any of these diseases.

After you've gathered this information and recorded it in your Family Health Diary, look for any patterns that emerge.

Obesity Let us assume that all four grandparents are still living and you've interviewed each of them. One of your grandparents is overweight and had a sibling who was overweight. That's a pattern of obesity in your side of the family. Now, suppose the same pattern emerges in your spouse's family, and further, you and your spouse are both struggling to keep your weight down. You now have evidence that your child will be at risk for obesity: a history of obesity on one or both sides of your child's family indicates that there is a genetic predisposition.

What do you do now? Take the measurements outlined below more often than normally recommended and intervene as soon as the rate of weight gain begins to accelerate. If your child is an adolescent, sit down and discuss the problem with him. Tell him he may be at increased risk of obesity and ask him to read the Family Medical Diary. Let him know that you're encouraging a pattern of healthy eating and exercise, and you're doing it before he begins to show any evidence of becoming obese.

Heart Disease, High Blood Pressure, Hypertension, and Diabetes Now suppose that your Family Health Diary indicates a clear history of heart disease (sometimes fatal at a young age) on one or both sides of the family. This will call for some careful detective work. Does anyone in the family also have a history of stroke, suggesting that high blood pressure could be the cause? Is there a history of diabetes (high blood sugar)? How about obesity? Were the cholesterol levels high? Did that family member smoke? These are all risk factors for heart attacks, so it is important to get as much specific information as possible.

What about you? Do you know your blood pressure readings, your cholesterol numbers, and your blood sugar? Are you overweight? All of these factors are important in deciding just how rigorous you'll have to be in employing dietary and exercise techniques during pregnancy and with your infant, toddler, school-age child, and adolescent. If a clear history of hypertension emerges, you'll want to be even more vigilant about limiting sodium and avoiding obesity. And if a clear history of diabetes emerges, again this means obesity must be avoided. Type II diabetes is now being reported in increasing numbers of obese children and adolescents. As you now know, obesity in childhood can play a direct role in heart disease and an indirect role in increasing the risk of hypertension, diabetes, and high cholesterol—three other direct causes of heart attacks.

If your family health history shows a pattern of heart disease, it clearly becomes important for your child to be both monitored for and protected from those factors that are direct causes of heart attacks. And it's important that you, as the parents, also are assessed for these factors.

Blood pressure should be monitored more often in children with family health histories of heart attacks. If your child becomes obese, her blood-sugar levels should be determined and the obesity treated according to your child's age and stage of development. As your child reaches adolescence, it is vital that you tell her that smoking (itself a major risk factor for heart attacks) is particularly detrimental to her health.

How about levels of cholesterol and other lipids? Some physicians feel that all children should have their serum cholesterol determined, but most do not think this is necessary. (See The Testing, below.) If a child has a strong family history of heart disease there is no doubt that a series of blood tests to determine total cholesterol—LDL (bad) cholesterol, HDL (good) cholesterol, and other lipids (triglycerides) should be done before age three. These tests are simple and can be done by a single finger prick. If the tests are abnormal, it's recommended that you feed your child a diet low in saturated fats. No more than 30 percent of daily calories (or no less than 20 percent) should come from fats—10 percent saturated and trans fats, 10 percent polyunsaturated, and 10 percent monounsaturated. In fact, all children at around ages four or five should follow this low-fat protocol. (These tests should be repeated yearly, and if they remain high, a more stringent fat-restriction program may be in order.)

Osteoporosis Finally, is there a history of osteoporosis in your family? Have there been hip or wrist fractures in older members, particularly the women? If so, your child must be considered at risk for this disease in later life. This is particularly true for girls, who are ten times as likely to develop osteoporosis as boys. Unfortunately, there is no test that can be done to confirm this extra risk. Bone density tests involve radiation (we certainly don't want to expose our children routinely to radiation) and must be done serially in adults to be of value. In addition, there are no normal values for children at any age. That makes your family health history even more important in determining risk.

Once this history is assembled you can decide whether your child falls into the high-risk category. If she does, than the preventative measures remain the same as for all children. You want her to build bones that are as strong as possible. Calcium is the key, but avoiding phosphorous-laden sodas is also important. Since calcium absorption is greatest from breast milk, if possible, children at risk should be breast-fed.

Finally, any weight-bearing exercise—such as jogging, jumping, running—is important, as it stimulates bone growth. All children should be encouraged to take these recommendations seriously, especially those at genetic risk for osteoporosis.

GATHERING INFORMATION To start off, take a look at the Family Health Tree. This tree targets the chronic disease history of your immediate family. Once you familiarize yourself with the Tree, begin to collect as much health information as possible from each family member to be included in the Family Health Diary and Medical Work Sheet that follow.

Family Health Tree

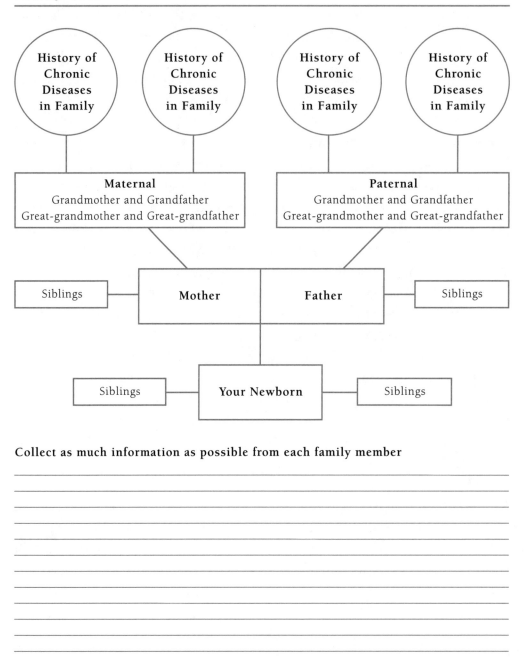

Collect as much information as possible from each family member

Family Medical Diary

Child's Name: Age:

MOTHER	FATHER
Name _____	Name _____
Age _____	Age _____
Ethnicity_____	Ethnicity _____
Date of Birth _____	Date of Birth _____
Weight/Height _____BMI_____	Weight/Height _____BMI_____
Cholesterol _____	Cholesterol _____
LDL_____	LDL _____
HDL _____	HDL _____
Blood Pressure _____	Blood Pressure _____
Smoke_____How Long_____	Smoke_____How Long_____

Known Ailments / Treatment

Heart Disease _____

_____

High Blood Pressure _____

_____

Type 2 Diabetes_____

_____

Cancer _____

_____

Osteoporosis _____

Other Known Ailments_____

_____

_____

_____

_____

Known Ailments / Treatment

Heart Disease _____

_____

High Blood Pressure _____

_____

Type 2 Diabetes _____

_____

Cancer _____

_____

Osteoporosis _____

Other Known Ailments_____

_____

_____

_____

_____

MATERNAL GRANDMOTHER

Name _____

Age _____

Ethnicity_____

Date of Birth _____

Weight/Height _____ BMI_____

Cholesterol _____

  LDL_____

  HDL _____

Blood Pressure _____

Smoke_____How Long_____

Known Ailments / Treatment

Heart Disease _____

_____

High Blood Pressure _____

_____

Type 2 Diabetes_____

_____

Cancer _____

_____

Osteoporosis _____

Height Loss _____

Bone Density_____

History of Fractures_____

_____

Other Known Ailments_____

_____

_____

_____

_____

PATERNAL GRANDMOTHER

Name _____

Age _____

Ethnicity _____

Date of Birth _____

Weight/Height _____ BMI _____

Cholesterol _____

  LDL _____

  HDL _____

Blood Pressure _____

Smoke_____How Long_____

Known Ailments / Treatment

Heart Disease _____

_____

High Blood Pressure _____

_____

Type 2 Diabetes _____

_____

Cancer _____

_____

Osteoporosis _____

Height Loss _____

Bone Density_____

History of Fractures_____

_____

Other Known Ailments_____

_____

_____

_____

_____

MATERNAL GRANDFATHER

Name _____

Age _____

Ethnicity_____

Date of Birth _____

Weight/Height _____BMI_____

Cholesterol _____

  LDL_____

  HDL _____

Blood Pressure _____

Smoke_____How Long_____

Known Ailments / Treatment

Heart Disease _____

_____

High Blood Pressure _____

_____

Type 2 Diabetes_____

_____

Cancer _____

_____

Osteoporosis_____

Height Loss _____

Bone Density_____

History of Fractures_____

_____

Other Known Ailments_____

_____

_____

_____

_____

PATERNAL GRANDFATHER

Name _____

Age _____

Ethnicity _____

Date of Birth _____

Weight/Height _____BMI _____

Cholesterol _____

  LDL _____

  HDL_____

Blood Pressure _____

Smoke_____How Long_____

Known Ailments / Treatment

Heart Disease _____

_____

High Blood Pressure _____

_____

Type 2 Diabetes _____

_____

Cancer _____

_____

Osteoporosis_____

Height Loss _____

Bone Density_____

History of Fractures_____

_____

Other Known Ailments_____

_____

_____

_____

_____

MATERNAL GREAT-GRANDMOTHER

Name _____

Age _____

Ethnicity_____

Date of Birth _____

Weight/Height _____BMI_____

Cholesterol _____

  LDL_____

  HDL _____

Blood Pressure _____

Smoke _____How Long_____

Known Ailments / Treatment

Heart Disease _____

_____

High Blood Pressure _____

_____

Type 2 Diabetes_____

_____

Cancer _____

_____

Osteoporosis _____

Height Loss _____

Bone Density_____

History of Fractures_____

_____

Other Known Ailments_____

_____

_____

_____

_____

PATERNAL GREAT-GRANDMOTHER

Name _____

Age _____

Ethnicity _____

Date of Birth _____

Weight/Height _____BMI _____

Cholesterol _____

  LDL _____

  HDL _____

Blood Pressure _____

Smoke _____How Long_____

Known Ailments / Treatment

Heart Disease _____

_____

High Blood Pressure _____

_____

Type 2 Diabetes _____

_____

Cancer _____

_____

Osteoporosis _____

Height Loss _____

Bone Density_____

History of Fractures_____

_____

Other Known Ailments_____

_____

_____

_____

_____

MATERNAL GREAT-GRANDFATHER

Name _____

Age _____

Ethnicity_____

Date of Birth _____

Weight/Height _____BMI_____

Cholesterol _____

   LDL_____

   HDL _____

Blood Pressure _____

Smoke_____How Long_____

Known Ailments / Treatment

Heart Disease _____

_____

High Blood Pressure _____

_____

Type 2 Diabetes_____

_____

Cancer _____

_____

Osteoporosis_____

Height Loss _____

Bone Density_____

History of Fractures_____

_____

Other Known Ailments_____

_____

_____

_____

_____

PATERNAL GREAT-GRANDFATHER

Name _____

Age _____

Ethnicity _____

Date of Birth _____

Weight/Height _____BMI _____

Cholesterol _____

   LDL _____

   HDL _____

Blood Pressure _____

Smoke_____How Long_____

Known Ailments / Treatment

Heart Disease _____

_____

High Blood Pressure _____

_____

Type 2 Diabetes _____

_____

Cancer _____

_____

Osteoporosis_____

Height Loss _____

Bone Density_____

History of Fractures_____

_____

Other Known Ailments_____

_____

_____

_____

_____

MATERNAL SIBLING

Name _____

Age _____

Ethnicity_____

Date of Birth _____

Weight/Height _____BMI_____

Cholesterol _____

  LDL_____

  HDL _____

Blood Pressure _____

Smoke _____How Long_____

Known Ailments / Treatment

Heart Disease _____

_____

High Blood Pressure _____

_____

Type 2 Diabetes_____

_____

Cancer _____

_____

Osteoporosis _____

Height Loss _____

Bone Density_____

History of Fractures_____

_____

Other Known Ailments_____

_____

_____

_____

_____

PATERNAL SIBLING

Name _____

Age _____

Ethnicity _____

Date of Birth _____

Weight/Height _____BMI_____

Cholesterol _____

  LDL _____

  HDL _____

Blood Pressure _____

Smoke _____How Long_____

Known Ailments / Treatment

Heart Disease _____

_____

High Blood Pressure _____

_____

Type 2 Diabetes _____

_____

Cancer _____

_____

Osteoporosis _____

Height Loss _____

Bone Density_____

History of Fractures_____

_____

Other Known Ailments_____

_____

_____

_____

_____

MATERNAL GRANDMOTHER'S SIBLING

Name _____

Age _____

Ethnicity_____

Date of Birth _____

Weight/Height _____BMI_____

Cholesterol _____

  LDL_____

  HDL _____

Blood Pressure _____

Smoke _____How Long_____

Known Ailments / Treatment

Heart Disease _____

_____

High Blood Pressure _____

_____

Type 2 Diabetes_____

_____

Cancer _____

_____

Osteoporosis _____

Height Loss _____

Bone Density_____

History of Fractures_____

_____

Other Known Ailments_____

_____

_____

_____

_____

PATERNAL GRANDMOTHER'S SIBLING

Name _____

Age _____

Ethnicity _____

Date of Birth _____

Weight/Height _____BMI _____

Cholesterol _____

  LDL _____

  HDL _____

Blood Pressure _____

Smoke _____How Long_____

Known Ailments / Treatment

Heart Disease _____

_____

High Blood Pressure _____

_____

Type 2 Diabetes _____

_____

Cancer _____

_____

Osteoporosis _____

Height Loss _____

Bone Density_____

History of Fractures_____

_____

Other Known Ailments_____

_____

_____

_____

_____

MATERNAL GRANDFATHER'S SIBLING

PATERNAL GRANDFATHER'S SIBLING

Name _____

Name _____

Age _____

Age _____

Ethnicity_____

Ethnicity_____

Date of Birth _____

Date of Birth _____

Weight/Height _____BMI_____

Weight/Height _____BMI_____

Cholesterol _____

Cholesterol _____

  LDL_____

  LDL_____

  HDL_____

  HDL_____

Blood Pressure _____

Blood Pressure _____

Smoke_____How Long_____

Smoke_____How Long_____

Known Ailments / Treatment

Known Ailments / Treatment

Heart Disease _____

Heart Disease _____

High Blood Pressure _____

High Blood Pressure _____

Type 2 Diabetes_____

Type 2 Diabetes_____

Cancer _____

Cancer _____

Osteoporosis_____

Osteoporosis_____

Height Loss _____

Height Loss _____

Bone Density_____

Bone Density_____

History of Fractures_____

History of Fractures_____

Other Known Ailments_____

Other Known Ailments_____

CHILD'S SIBLING

Name _____

Age _____

Ethnicity_____

Date of Birth _____

Birth Weight _____

Birth Height_____

Breast or Bottle Fed _____

  How Long _____

Age Solid Foods Introduced_____

Age Milk Introduced   Whole _____

                              Skim _____

Allergies _____

_____

_____

_____

_____

Notes _____

_____

_____

_____

_____

CHILD'S SIBLING

Name _____

Age _____

Ethnicity _____

Date of Birth _____

Birth Weight _____

Birth Height _____

Breast- or Bottle-Fed _____

  How Long _____

Age Solid Foods Introduced_____

Age Milk Introduced   Whole _____

                              Skim _____

Allergies _____

_____

_____

_____

_____

Notes _____

_____

_____

_____

_____

THE TESTING We're so lucky to be living in an age of advanced medical testing. Today, we have everything from blood tests to MRI's that weren't conceivable even a few years ago. By using the family medical history as a tool and having certain tests performed, we can now predict which children may be potentially at risk for certain adult diseases. While these children may not need any special treatment, they may well need more attention focused on their diet. This is disease intervention at its best.

Here are four common tests than can help you and your doctor identify your child's risk for developing obesity or chronic disease.

- At each visit, your doctor will measure weight and height or length to be sure that your child is growing normally and that the rate of weight gain does not change.

- As your child gets older, a blood pressure measurement should become part of every physical exam. If blood pressure is too high, that means there may be too much salt in your child's diet.

- If your child needs an X-ray for any reason, take this opportunity to ask the radiologist to assess your child's bone density. These test results could indicate a need for more calcium in your child's diet.

- A blood sugar test is not necessary if your child is not obese. If, on the other hand, your child is obese, then a blood sugar test should be done, since Type II diabetes has become so common among obese children, especially adolescents.

Dr. W

Imagine pricking a child's finger, taking a drop of blood, and being able to assess which disease the child is at high risk for developing in middle and old age. In some cases this may be possible, in most it is not. For example, we could test all children for the various types of cholesterol carried in the blood. We could then see if the levels were "normal" for the child's age or if they are too high. Some pediatricians advocate this approach, but most believe that this should not be done on every child. The treatment is the same regardless of the level of the child's cholesterol: a diet in which 20 to 30 percent of calories come from fat and an increase in their activity. So rather than testing serum cholesterol in all children, we recommend that it be tested only in children with a family history that puts them in a high-risk category. This test should be done around age three or four to establish a baseline and then repeated annually to find out if the diet that has been introduced is having any effect. Incidentally, do you, as parents, know your cholesterol level? If you don't, find out—for your child's sake and for your own.

Medical Work Sheet [page 1]

Insurance Provider_____

Policy #_____

Child's Name _____ Date of Birth_____

Birth Weight _____ Birth Height_____

Breast- or Bottle-Fed _____ How Long _____

Age Solid Foods Introduced _____

Age Milk Introduced: Whole Milk_____ Skim Milk _____

Siblings:

Birth Weight _____ Birth Length _____

Birth Weight _____ Birth Length _____

Birth Weight _____ Birth Length _____

Health Care Information

	Doctor's Name	Specialty	Address	Phone/E-mail
Primary Pediatrician				
Specialist				
Specialist				
Specialist				

Medical Conditions

Condition/Diagnosis	Date of Onset	Date of Recovery	Details

Medical Work Sheet (page 2)

Allergies – Description

_____

_____

_____

_____

_____

_____

_____

Prescription Medications

Drug Name	Dosage/How often	Reasons for Taking	When Discontinued

Notes

_____

_____

_____

_____

_____

_____

15

Creating Your Child's Growth Book from Newborn to Adolescent—Tracking Height and Weight

The best way to evaluate whether your child is getting too many, too few, or just the right number of calories, and thus gaining weight at a healthy and appropriate rate, is to create a Growth Book that tracks the changes in your child's height and weight. This way, whenever you notice significant shifts in percentiles (when the line that represents your child's weight makes a sudden or sharp upward movement), you'll be able to make the nutritional and activity changes necessary to prevent your child from potentially becoming obese. This one simple act can have a profound effect on your child's life, since, as we now know, obesity invariably leads to a future laden with chronic diseases.

Your Growth Book will allow you to gather a clear picture of your child's physical development, from infancy through adolescence. Keeping a Growth Book allows you to become a partner with your pediatrician, as you record important information that can be passed along to him or her at your visits. After visits, you'll add the information you receive from your pediatrician to the Growth Book. Be sure to tell your pediatrician about any changes you see in between scheduled visits.

Measuring Your Child's Height and Weight

During the first year, when you're seeing your pediatrician at frequent intervals, you don't need to take any measurements yourself. The doctor will take the measurements, and you can record them on your own charts. After your visits become less frequent, you can take height and weight measurements every few months. Once your child starts school, take the measurements every six months. If height and weight are increasing at the same rate, don't measure more often—you don't want your child to overly fixate on weight. But if weight begins to increase faster than height, then it may be time to start cutting back on calories and increase your child's exercise. If the weight gain continues, call your physician.

When your child is young, while bathing or changing her, you can use a tape measure to calculate her length. To weigh her at home, first step on the scale, weigh yourself, and record the number. Then hold her in your arms and step back onto the scale. Subtract your weight (the first number) from the weight of you and your baby (the sec-

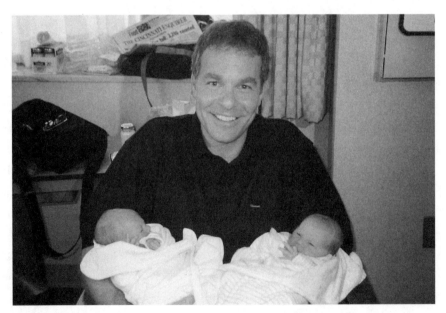

Daddy Jeff is 6'4". It will be fun tracking Max's and Kate's growth.

ond number) to calculate your baby's weight. Plot that number on the Growth Chart for your child's age and gender.

Once your baby is walking, you can treat measuring as a fun activity. Hang a measuring tape from a door or wall, and mark your child's height. This way, everyone in the family can celebrate your toddler's growth. To weigh your toddler, purchase a scale with large digital numbers and let your toddler weigh herself as you watch. (She'll also get a head start in learning numbers and circumvent the fear of scales!)

We've provided you with a sample chart to get you started. You'll notice two separate sets of growth lines. The lower set of lines represents what incremental increases in a child's weight might look like. The upper lines in this sample chart signify incremental increases in height or stature. These lines allow you to see what percentile your child falls into. They must be considered together in order to determine whether your child is at a healthy weight or is overweight.

So let's say your child is growing in the sixtieth percentile for her height, and the sixtieth percentile for her weight. That's fine. But if at some point you notice when you measure your child that she falls into the sixtieth percentile for height, but now falls into the seventieth percentile for weight, that could signify a potential problem. And if the next time you check her weight, if it then jumps to the eightieth percentile, you need to be aware that your child is in danger of becoming obese. Once again, it doesn't matter which percentile your child falls into—the sixtieth percentile simply means that forty percent of all children are taller or heavier, and sixty percent are shorter or lighter— what matters is that the percentile for both height *and* weight remain constant. We have to remember, though, that every child is different—some are short and stocky, some are petite, and others are tall and lean. That's why you may find that your child falls into two different percentiles for height and weight (ie, the seventieth percentile for height, and the seventy-fifth percentile for weight). Again, that in itself is not a problem, as long as the percentiles remain constant.

It bears repeating. *As soon as your child's weight starts accelerating faster than her height, she could be moving towards obesity.*

Now it's time to familiarize yourself with our sample chart, so that you can begin to plot your own child's development. You'll quickly see that you're not just plotting numbers, but the actual growth of your child.

SAMPLE BOYS GROWTH CHART
2 TO 18 YEARS

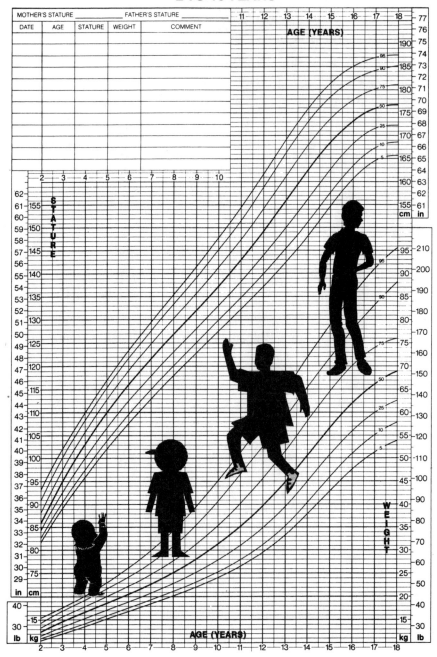

GIRLS GROWTH CHART
BIRTH TO 36 MONTHS

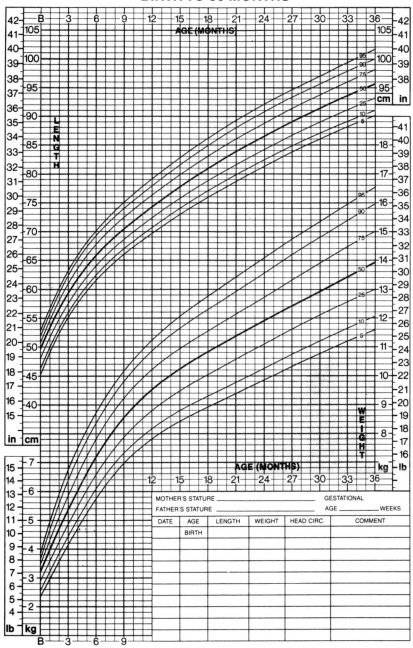

BOYS GROWTH CHART
BIRTH TO 36 MONTHS

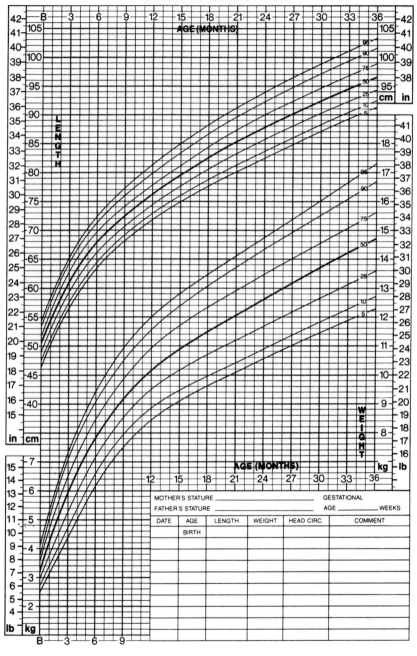

GIRLS GROWTH CHART
2 TO 18 YEARS

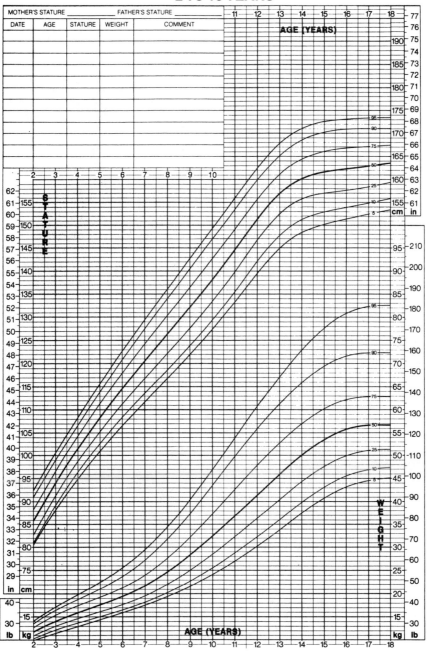

BOYS GROWTH CHART
2 TO 18 YEARS

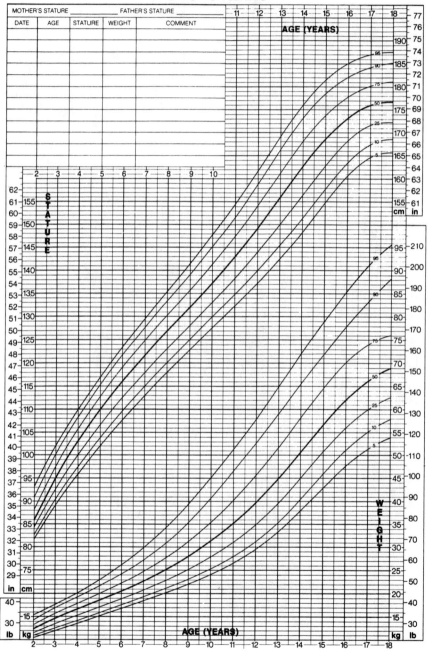

Calculating Your Child's BMI

Since 2000, the pediatric community has been using a new children's BMI formula that measures girls against girls and boys against boys. Doctors use BMI charts when they notice that a child's weight is increasing faster than her height. If you're concerned about your child's weight, discuss it with your pediatrician and ask if a baseline BMI should be taken. After the doctor does the initial baseline BMI, you can then plot that calculation on your child's BMI chart (below). As your child gets older and doctor visits become less frequent, you can do your own calculations to track how your child compares to other children in the same age range, if you think your child is gaining too much weight. But please remember—although you want to avoid obesity, you don't want your child to become obsessive about his or her weight.

To calculate your child's BMI, use this formula: (Don't let it scare you!)

$$\text{BMI} = \left(\frac{\text{Weight in Pounds}}{(\text{Height in Inches}) \times (\text{Height in Inches})} \right) \times 703$$

To better understand how the formula works, let's go through the calculations.

A child who is 33 inches tall and weighs 39 pounds:

1. Multiply his height in inches by his height in inches—33 × 33 = 1089
2. Now divide his pounds by his height times height + 39 divided by 1089 = 0.358
3. Next multiply 0.358 by 703 = 25.2
4. That child's BMI is 25.2

After you've calculated your child's BMI, plot it on the BMI graph that follows. This will tell you if your child is overweight for his or her age.

If you have a computer, you can simplify this calculation by going to http://www.cdc.gov/nccbphp/cnpa/bmip-means.htm. Just type in your child's height and weight—they'll do all the calculations for you and give you the correct BMI.

Children's Calculated Body Mass Index — Heights: 29"—43" Weights: 35 lbs.—43 lbs.

Whenever a child's specific height or weight measurement is not listed, round to the closest number on the table

Height		Weight Kg	15.9	16.1	16.3	16.6	16.8	17.0	17.2	17.5	17.7	17.9	18.1	18.4	18.6	18.8	19.1	19.3	19.5
		Lb	35	35.5	36	36.5	37	37.5	38	38.5	39	39.5	40	40.5	41	41.5	42	42.5	43
Cm	In																		
73.7	29		29.3	29.7	30.1	30.5	30.9	31.3	31.8	32.2	32.6	33.0	33.4	33.9	34.3	34.7			
74.9	29.5		28.3	28.7	29.1	29.5	29.9	30.3	30.7	31.1	31.5	31.9	32.3	32.7	33.1	33.5	33.9	34.3	34.7
76.2	30		27.3	27.7	28.1	28.5	28.9	29.3	29.7	30.1	30.5	30.9	31.2	31.6	32.0	32.4	32.8	33.2	33.6
77.5	30.5		26.5	26.8	27.2	27.6	28.0	28.3	28.7	29.1	29.5	29.9	30.2	30.6	31.0	31.4	31.7	32.1	32.5
78.7	31		25.6	26.0	26.3	26.7	27.1	27.4	27.8	28.2	28.5	28.9	29.3	29.6	30.0	30.4	30.7	31.1	31.5
80.0	31.5		24.8	25.2	25.5	25.9	26.2	26.6	26.9	27.3	27.6	28.0	28.3	28.7	29.1	29.4	29.8	30.1	30.5
81.3	32		24.0	24.4	24.7	25.1	25.4	25.7	26.1	26.4	26.8	27.1	27.5	27.8	28.2	28.5	28.8	29.2	29.5
82.6	32.5		23.3	23.6	24.0	24.3	24.6	25.0	25.3	25.6	26.0	26.3	26.6	27.0	27.3	27.6	28.0	28.3	28.6
83.8	33		22.6	22.9	23.2	23.6	23.9	24.2	24.5	24.9	25.2	25.5	25.8	26.1	26.5	26.8	27.1	27.4	27.8
85.1	33.5		21.9	22.2	22.6	22.9	23.2	23.5	23.8	24.1	24.4	24.7	25.1	25.4	25.7	26.0	26.3	26.6	26.9
86.4	34		21.3	21.6	21.9	22.2	22.5	22.8	23.1	23.4	23.7	24.0	24.3	24.6	24.9	25.5	25.5	25.8	26.2
87.6	34.5		20.7	21.0	21.3	21.6	21.9	22.2	22.4	22.7	23.0	23.3	23.6	23.9	24.2	24.5	24.8	25.1	25.4
88.9	35		20.1	20.4	20.7	20.9	21.2	21.5	21.8	22.1	22.4	22.7	23.0	23.2	23.5	23.8	24.1	24.4	24.7
90.2	35.5		19.5	19.8	20.1	20.4	20.6	20.9	21.2	21.5	21.8	22.0	22.3	22.6	22.9	23.2	23.4	23.7	24.0
91.4	36		19.0	19.3	19.5	19.8	20.1	20.3	20.6	20.9	21.2	21.4	21.7	22.0	22.2	22.5	22.8	23.1	23.3
92.7	36.5		18.5	18.7	19.0	19.3	19.5	19.8	20.1	20.3	20.6	20.8	21.1	21.4	21.6	21.9	22.2	22.4	22.7
94.0	37		18.0	18.2	18.5	18.7	19.0	19.3	19.5	19.8	20.0	20.3	20.5	20.8	21.1	21.3	21.6	21.8	22.1
95.3	37.5		17.5	17.7	18.0	18.2	18.5	18.7	19.0	19.2	19.5	19.7	20.0	20.2	20.5	20.7	21.0	21.2	21.5
96.5	38		17.0	17.3	17.5	17.8	18.0	18.3	18.5	18.7	19.0	19.2	19.5	19.7	20.0	20.2	20.4	20.7	20.9
97.8	38.5		16.6	16.8	17.1	17.3	17.6	17.8	18.0	18.3	18.5	18.7	19.0	19.2	19.4	19.7	19.9	20.2	20.4
99.1	39		16.2	16.4	16.6	16.9	17.1	17.3	17.6	17.8	18.0	18.3	18.5	18.7	19.0	19.2	19.4	19.6	19.9
100.3	39.5		15.8	16.0	16.2	16.4	16.7	16.9	17.1	17.3	17.6	17.8	18.0	18.2	18.5	18.7	18.9	19.2	19.4
101.6	40		15.4	15.6	15.8	16.0	16.3	16.5	16.7	16.9	17.1	17.4	17.6	17.8	18.0	18.2	18.5	18.7	18.9
102.9	40.5		15.0	15.2	15.4	15.6	15.9	16.1	16.3	16.5	16.7	16.9	17.1	17.4	17.6	17.8	18.0	18.2	18.4
104.1	41		14.6	14.8	15.1	15.3	15.5	15.7	15.9	16.1	16.3	16.5	16.7	16.9	17.1	17.4	17.6	17.8	18.0
105.4	41.5		14.3	14.5	14.7	14.9	15.1	15.3	15.5	15.7	15.9	16.1	16.3	16.5	16.7	16.9	17.1	17.3	17.6
106.7	42		13.9	14.1	14.3	14.5	14.7	14.9	15.1	15.3	15.5	15.7	15.9	16.1	16.3	16.5	16.7	16.9	17.1
108.0	42.5		13.6	13.8	14.0	14.2	14.4	14.6	14.8	15.0	15.2	15.4	15.6	15.8	16.0	16.2	16.3	16.5	16.7
109.2	43		13.3	13.5	13.7	13.9	14.1	14.3	14.4	14.6	14.8	15.0	15.2	15.4	15.6	15.8	16.0	16.2	16.4

16

When You Visit Your Pediatrician—a Checklist

When my twins, Kate and Max, were born, I was a mom again at fifty-two. It had been years since I had made a "baby" visit to my pediatrician. What were those questions I should ask? What questions were other mothers asking? One thing I did remember was that the appointment would go a lot smoother if I thought about my questions and made a checklist in advance, rather than trying to remember while I had babies wiggling and possibly peeing all over me. Dr. Winick has helped us prepare a checklist of commonly asked questions for parents to ask their pediatrician.

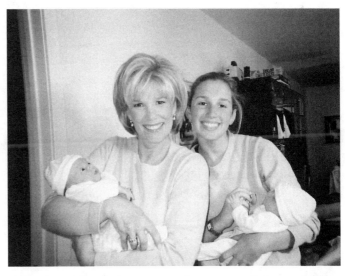

Big sister Lindsay helps Mom get the twins ready for a trip to the doctor.

Dr. W *Most mothers, especially new mothers, want to know if they're asking their pediatricians the right questions. Like you, they want to expand their conversations with their pediatricians to be sure they're covering all their baby's health essentials. As a parent myself—and now a proud grandparent!—I know that you want to get the best from your child's pediatrician. That's why it's important to know that your baby will be best served by first informing your pediatrician of your family's health history. The more inclusive the history, the more information your pediatrician will have at his or her disposal for your child's medical treatment.*

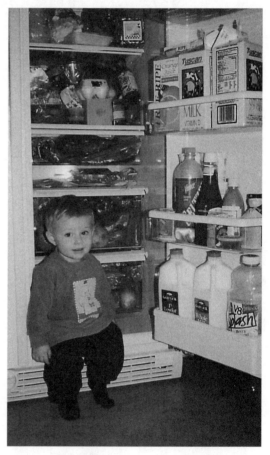

So, which questions should you ask on each visit to your pediatrician? Take a look at the list that follows and know that there are no set answers to these questions, nor are these the only questions to ask. Use them as a guide, and as you think of them, add more to your own checklist. After you get the answers, record them in your Family Medical Diary and on your child's Growth Charts. Remember, when your children are healthy, grown adults, they'll be able to pass this information along to their children and their children's children. It's a tradition you want to promote.

As a doting and concerned grandfather, I'm trying to steer Grandson Bradley in the right direction

Commonly Asked Questions for Your Checklist

1. *How much should my baby be eating? How can I tell if my baby is getting enough milk?*

2. *Does my baby need water to drink as well as breast milk or formula?*

3. *Is it possible to overfeed my baby?*

4. *Does my infant need fluoride drops?*

5. *I've heard that iron is constipating. Is it safe to use formula without iron?*

6. *When do I need to start giving my baby more than just milk?*

7. *Which foods should I give my baby?*

8. *What is my baby's height, weight, and what percentile does he fall into for each?*

9. *My baby's food seems tasteless. Is it okay to add salt or sugar?*

10. *I've heard infants sleep through the night better if you give them solids. Can I add cereal to my baby's bottle?*

11. *Should I cut down on my baby's milk when he starts eating solid food?*

12. *At what age can my baby start juice? What kind and how much?*

13. *Can I give my eight-month-old child a bottle in the crib?*

14. *I'm a vegan. Can I raise my baby as a vegan too?*

15. *When can I start giving my baby cow's milk?*

16. *My toddler only likes a few foods and sometimes hardly eats at all. Should I worry?*

17. *My child doesn't eat at his meals. Could I be giving him too much milk or juice?*

18. *My husband and I are on a low-fat diet, when can I place my child on this diet?*

19. My husband and I have a history of early heart disease. Should my child have any special tests? If so, what kind and at what age?

20. If my child is lactose intolerant and consumes no dairy foods, should she take a calcium supplement?

21. How can I tell if my child is fat? Should I put my child on a diet?

22. How should I feed my child when he is sick?

23. How many sodas are okay for my child?

24. My child seems hungry throughout the day. Is it okay if my child snacks? What should the snacks be?

25. My child is playing sports. Does she have different nutritional needs?

17

An R~x~ for Your Sick Child

Whether your child is fighting off a bacterial or viral infection, stomach ailments (diarrhea or vomiting), an injury, or recuperating from surgery, providing a nutritionally sound diet is an essential part of a recovery program. Your pediatrician may need to be consulted, depending upon the nature of the illness or injury, but here are some general guidelines that Dr. Winick recommends. As a parent, it's imperative that you remember one cardinal rule: *when in doubt, call your physician.*

Dr.W **Acute Bacterial Infections**

Children are prone to bacterial infections of all types, which include tonsillitis, ear infections, boils, and abscessed teeth. (Pneumonia, bronchitis, croup, and infections of the urinary tract, though much less common, are usually much more serious.) All bacterial infections should be properly diagnosed and specifically treated, usually with antibiotics.

Fever

One of the body's major defense mechanisms against bacterial infection is fever. The body temperature rises from 98.6 degrees Fahrenheit often to 101 degrees Fahrenheit or higher, and poses an added strain on your child's body. Any child who has fever is burning calories less efficiently than he should. Some calories available for normal body function are diverted to keep the temperature elevated. That means when your child has a fever, he or she needs more calories. (The old adage that urges you to "starve a fever" is bad advice.) Find foods your child likes to eat: Ice cream, milk shakes, and puddings are all high in calories and usually kid favorites.

While your child is sick, don't worry about a perfectly balanced diet. You can make up for those missing nutrients by offering him or her a multivitamin and multimineral supplement during and after the illness. The B vitamins are particularly important at this time because they are crucial for the production of energy from the carbohydrates in food. (Remember, extra vitamins are of little value unless you also provide adequate calories.)

Dehydration

Along with fever, parents need to be concerned with dehydration. As the body temperature rises, more water and certain minerals are lost through the skin in the sweat. To replace them, encourage your child to drink juice, lemonade, tea, and soup. Clearly, grandmother's chicken soup was, and still is, a good choice. It provides water, minerals, and vitamins in the broth and calories from the fat.

Recuperation

When your child is recuperating from an acute illness with fever, there are certain other nutritional principles you should bear in mind. As your child's temperature returns to normal and the illness begins to subside, her caloric requirements will drop. Since she'll still be in bed, she'll be much less active than usual. Remember, her appetite will probably have returned and the temptation to overfeed her will be irresistible. Resist! Don't overfeed her, especially if the convalescent phase is going to be more than a few days.

Protein is very important at this time. During the acute phase of your child's illness, tissue protein breaks down, slowing down normal growth. While he or she is recuperating, replace the high-calorie, high-fat ice cream and milk shakes with lower-calorie, higher-protein chicken, fish, turkey, or beef to restimulate growth.

Calcium balance is also important, especially if a period of prolonged bed rest (one or more weeks) is necessary. Sustained bed rest causes bones to lose calcium at a faster rate than usual. So if your child must be in bed for a week or more, encourage him to eat foods high in calcium (see chapter 7). If he refuses to eat these foods, then a calcium supplement (500 mg/daily) is recommended.

Acute Viral Infections

Although most children have been immunized against the more serious acute viral infections, viral disease still constitutes one of the most common ills of childhood.

Influenza, for example, can incapacitate a child for several weeks. Though antibiotics are prescribed for bacterial diseases, there is no specific therapy at present for viral diseases. The body's own defense mechanisms will have to do the healing. That's why nutritional support is even more important for viral infections. Proper nutrition during this period will help those defense mechanisms function most efficiently. As with bacterial infections, your child will need adequate calories, plenty of fluids, and supplementary vitamins and minerals.

If the illness lasts more than a week, foods rich in calcium, or a calcium supplement are recommended.

Gastroenteritis (Diarrhea and Vomiting)

Diarrhea is one of the most common afflictions of young children. It may vary from an occasional loose bowel movement to explosive liquid stools that continue for days and sometimes for weeks. If diarrhea persists in a young child, medical help should be sought. Sometimes the diarrhea may be due to an infection that will respond to specific treatment. Other times there is no specific treatment and the child must be supported nutritionally until the diarrhea subsides.

The chief aim of treatment is to replace the fluid and nutrients that are being lost in the stool without aggravating the diarrhea. The first rule is to allow the irritated bowel to rest as much as possible. This means that your child must be given foods that are as easily digested as possible. Simple sugars (apple juice, applesauce, Jell-O), which are easily digestible, are usually given first. In general, avoid giving him fats of any sort or proteins from meats or vegetables. Complex carbohydrates should be used sparingly as well.

Since fluid loss may be extensive, replenishing him with fluids containing electrolytes (dissolved minerals) is also recommended. Various easily available liquids are excellent for treating diarrhea in its early stages, such as diluted apple juice, flat ginger ale, or Pedialyte. Small amounts given frequently will usually work best, but consult your pediatrician. If the diarrhea begins to subside, you can continue this treatment for twenty-four hours and then slowly begin to add liquids that contain other nutrients. If your sick child is an infant on formula, a temporary change of formula may be necessary.

Recuperation

When the stool begins to take form, solid foods can gradually be reintroduced. Start with a food containing simple sugar, such as mashed apple or applesauce. Then slowly introduce foods with more complex carbohydrates, such as cooked cereal. If at any point the diarrhea reappears, withdraw that food and continue as before. Be patient. Reintroduce foods slowly, especially complex carbohydrates, fats, and foods high in protein.

Vomiting

When a child with diarrhea suddenly begins vomiting, you should seek medical help immediately. Nausea and vomiting may signal some dietary indiscretion, or they may be signs of a more serious underlying problem. Vomiting should not be confused with simple regurgitation, or spitting up. Many young infants will spit up after a feeding if they have had too much, if they have been fed too fast, or if they have not been properly burped. Occasionally a young infant may actually vomit significant amounts for the same reasons. Repeated vomiting, particularly forceful vomiting in an infant around three to six weeks of age (especially a firstborn male infant), may signal an abnormality of the muscle that allows the stomach to empty. This condition, called pyloric stenosis, must be corrected. A relatively simple surgical procedure is usually the best form of treatment.

In older children vomiting may be the first sign of a viral infection and may be accompanied by fever, headache, and a general sick feeling. If your child is suffering from this kind of viral infection, the vomiting is the first symptom that must be dealt with. If it is not brought under control, none of the other feeding measures suggested above can be undertaken. Often the child may be able to tolerate small amounts of concentrated calories in the form of simple sugars. During the era of soda fountains, cola syrup in small amounts fed by spoon was often good for this purpose. Today this is difficult to obtain. Fruit gelatin desserts and fruit syrups can be used in the same way.

Recuperation

Once the vomiting has subsided you can increase the quantity of these substances and include small amounts of carbohydrate solid foods, such as crackers or dry cereals. Don't use foods that are high in fat (dairy products) until the child is retaining food well. At this point the treatment becomes the same as for other viral infections.

If headache is a very prominent symptom and if the vomiting is very forceful, you should seek medical advice immediately. Although the symptoms may be the result of a simple viral infection, they may also be caused by other problems, which require specific treatment.

Your doctor may want to use medications to control the diarrhea or vomiting. This should not change your nutritional approach but may allow you to progress from one step to the next more rapidly.

Recovery from Surgery

Any surgery will put a major strain on the body. A certain amount of tissue destruction will have taken place, and proper healing and wound repair are necessary. Under these circumstances your child's nutritional requirements will increase. If the operation was associated with an acute illness such as appendicitis and your child has sustained a period of undernutrition before, during, and shortly after the operation, adequate calories should be supplied during convalescence. But since your child will be less active than usual, don't overdo it. Protein is very important. Tissue repair requires a good supply of amino acids, which are available as a result of eating generous amounts of protein. Foods high in vitamin C and vitamin C supplements (100 mg daily) have been shown to support wound healing. If prolonged bed rest is required, a calcium supplement is also recommended. Be sure to follow your doctor's advice carefully.

Injuries

Depending on the nature and severity of an injury, nutrition is a vital part of your child's recovery. Significant blood loss (a severe nosebleed or cut that has bled for a long time) can lead to iron deficiency and anemia. Iron supplementation may be recommended. If the bleeding has been sustained internally (a bruise or hematoma), then iron supplementation is not necessary, since the iron in the broken red blood cells will be reutilized by the body.

Burns

Burns may cause your child to lose protein. If your child suffers from a burn, and the skin and the layers just beneath have been badly damaged, a clear serumlike material will ooze out of the burned area, sometimes for several days, until a crust is formed. This material is composed mostly of protein. From a nutritional point of view, this means encouraging your child to eat foods high in protein such as meat, eggs, and fish.

Breaks and Fractures

Breaks and fractures also require nutritional backup. A simple fracture uses up a great deal of calcium during the healing process. When a bone is broken, it leaches calcium from other bones, which means that the fracture will heal partly at the expense of the other bones in the body, and overall calcium balance in the body will suffer. To avoid a calcium imbalance, add calcium-rich foods to your child's meals. Again, if your child is unwilling or unable to eat these foods, a calcium supplement may be recommended. Consult your pediatrician.

With more serious fractures that require a prolonged period in bed, the entire body is somewhat immobilized and the affected limb completely immobilized. Under these conditions, calcium is lost more rapidly, and a supplement (1 gram per day in an older child) is recommended. Avoid phosphorus-laden soft drinks. A high-phosphorus diet impairs calcium absorption.

Since all injuries involve a certain amount of tissue repair, adequate amounts of vitamin C should be consumed. As with surgery, a supplement containing 100 mg daily should be more than sufficient.

Pica

If your child, toddler age or above, actually craves nonedible substances and eats them, he or she has a serious problem called pica. Instances of consuming excessive amounts of dirt, clay, plaster, ashes, laundry starch, string, putty, paint chips, plaster, paper, crayons, and matches, among many other items, have all been reported.

The most dangerous aspect of pica is its frequent association with lead poisoning. Eating paint and plaster from older buildings in which leaded paint was used, or chewing on old batteries that contain lead can cause chronic lead poisoning, a very serious disease. It is currently estimated that 5 to 10 percent of children between the ages of one and five have some degree of lead poisoning, and about two hundred children die each year as a result of lead poisoning in the United States.

While pica has been associated with a variety of nutritional deficiencies including a vitamin C deficiency and a deficiency of calcium and vitamin D, the major nutritional consideration is iron deficiency. Some studies suggest that at least in some children, an iron deficiency actually causes pica. The theory (by no means proven) is that the child has a subconscious drive to seek iron and that his often bizarre consumption pattern is in response to that drive. Whatever the reason, children with severe pica have been cured by treating their iron deficiency with supplemental iron. If your child shows evidence of pica, make sure that he is not iron deficient. If in doubt, a few days of supplemental iron will do no harm and may diminish the pica.

If your doctor determines that lead levels in your child's blood are too high, he or she will decide on a specific treatment. But whatever the treatment decision—medication may be warranted—certain dietary modifications may help clear the blood of lead. A diet high in calcium and in phosphorus, plus extra vitamin D (no more than 400 IU) may promote the removal of lead from the blood, where it is potentially dangerous, into the bones, where it is harmless.

We hope that these nutritional guidelines for treating your sick child will help you as a parent to understand when to call a physician and why your doctor has suggested a certain treatment. If you don't understand, don't be afraid to ask questions. Understanding is the foundation upon which good treatment is built.

PART IV

The Recipes

Introduction

Learning what our bodies need in order to get and stay strong and disease free is an important part of the growing-up-healthy plan. But finding wholesome and tasty ways to incorporate nutritious ingredients into our daily lives is equally important, which is why I'm including a selection of my favorite nutritious recipes here.

Recently, my husband, Jeff, and I had the opportunity to visit my daughter Lindsay in Rome, where she was studying abroad. I couldn't help but notice that while Italians eat bread, olive oil, and pasta, they're thinner and live longer than us! As my daughters would say, "What's up with that?" A trip to an Italian grocery store quickly answered that question. As Lindsay pointed out, "You won't find an aisle of sugared cereal, processed chips, or cookies with ingredients that you can't pronounce, and you won't find an aisle of frozen TV dinners. The Italians use fresh ingredients, and instead of meat and pota-toes, they prepare meals with an abundance of fruits and vegetables." Lindsay also told me that when Italian kids come home from school, rather than snacking on that fine old American standby, a bologna sandwich, their moms make heart-healthy bruschetta for them, good Italian bread grilled with olive oil and topped with fresh chopped tomatoes, chopped onions, and basil. No wonder they learn to love healthy foods at an early age.

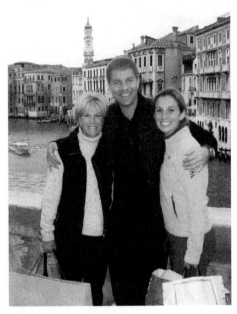

When Jeff and I visited Lindsay in Italy we couldn't help but notice that everything they serve is fresh and homemade.

I've looked for dishes that will encourage families with children of all ages to eat foods with healthy ingredients. I've kept all of you time-starved parents in mind too, and so have tried to make these recipes as easy and convenient as possible. That means some-times I'll refer you to frozen (or canned) ver-sions of ingredients. We all know we should use fresh vegetables whenever possible—Dr. Winick says he can't stress this enough!—but if the difference between frozen or fresh means the difference between a nourishing meal prepared at home or take-out fast food, please . . . use the frozen ingredients. Let's keep it simple. And let's keep it healthy.

In collecting these recipes I've tried to keep in mind the broad scope of this book, which is why I've included some delicious recipes for toddlers, and some for older children. Since these recipes weren't necessarily crafted for children in their first two years, when cooking for your toddler, please be sure that he or she has tried each ingredient separately before serving any dish. Now that we know we should be teaching our children to eat as little salt (sodium) as possible, always look for low-sodium varieties. When not available, drain and rinse regular canned products, which are usually high in salt. Also, be cautious when adding salt "to taste." Remember, your taste buds may scream for more salt, but that's not your child's taste preference, unless you make it that way. If there's a history of hypertension in your family, then you want to be especially diligent. In order to help you remember about the salt concern, we've added "optional" after every "salt to taste" direction.

You'll find all of these recipes easier if you plan meals ahead, keep a well-stocked pantry, and hopefully get your children involved with shopping and preparation. Your kids will be much more inclined to eat foods which they've had a hand in preparing, and you'll be laying down the groundwork for lifelong healthy eating habits. Remember, it's never too late to start growing up healthy.

18

Salads

Beets and Mandarin Oranges with Walnuts

This is the kind of dish we all love because it looks colorful, tastes delicious, is loaded with nutrients, and is a no-brainer to make. Your kids will love its sweetness and can even help you make it. It's so easy! This recipe serves 4 adult portions.

Ingredients

1 package vacuum-sealed cooked beets, or 1 15-oz can, or 6 fresh beets, cooked and peeled

1 small red onion, thinly sliced

1 T vegetable oil

2 T cider vinegar

¼ cup nonfat sour cream

Salt (optional) and pepper to taste

Boston or Bibb lettuce

½ cup mandarin oranges, drained

¼ cup chopped walnuts

Directions

1. Slice beets into julienne strips. Whisk oil and vinegar together, then toss with onions. Mix in the sour cream and season with salt (optional) and pepper to taste.

2. In a shallow bowl or on a serving platter, place the beets on top of a bed of soft lettuce leaves. Arrange mandarin orange slices around the edge of the leaves.

3. Sprinkle walnuts on top. Serve.

Carrot and Raisin Slaw

Kids always seem to like carrot salad; maybe it's the Bugs Bunny influence, I don't know. But carrots are a winning choice, consistently making the top of the list as a major disease fighter. They're loaded with the antioxidant beta-carotene, which boosts the immune system, protects our eyes, guards against cancer, and is even said to be crucial in learning and memory. So when your kids say, "What's up, Doc?" tell them Bugs's favorite carrot salad. Just make sure that the apple you choose is crisp, and not too sweet. (Granny Smith and Golden Delicious work well.) This recipe serves 4–6 adult portions.

Ingredients

1 10½-oz bag of grated carrots

2 medium-size apples, peeled and grated

1 cup plain yogurt

1 T honey

1 pinch of celery seeds

Juice of 1 lemon

⅓ cup raisins or dried currants

½ tsp salt (optional) and a dash of ground pepper

Option: ¼ cup toasted sunflower seeds, cashews, and almonds

Option: ¼ cup chopped pecans, toasted

Directions

1. In a large bowl, mix together the carrots, apples, and raisins (and sunflower seeds, cashews, almonds, if using).

2. Blend together yogurt, honey, celery seed, lemon juice, salt and pepper. Add to carrot-apple-raisin mixture.

3. Mix well and chill.

Chickpea, Carrot, and Parsley Salad

This recipe can be used as a salad or as a vegetarian main dish, served with warmed pita bread, sliced into wedges. It's delicious and nutritious and makes a beautiful presentation. This recipe serves 8 adult portions as a salad, or 4–6 as a main dish.

Ingredients

1 19-oz can chickpeas, drained and rinsed

1 cup loosely packed fresh, flat-leaf parsley, coarsely chopped

1 cup loosely packed shredded carrot

½ cup sliced radishes

½ cup chopped scallions, white and green parts

3 T fresh lemon juice

1 tsp ground coriander

Kosher salt (optional) and freshly ground black pepper

6 T extra-virgin olive oil

⅓ cup crumbled feta cheese or toasted pine nuts (optional)

Directions

1. In a mixing bowl, mash ½ cup of the chickpeas into a coarse paste with a potato masher or wooden spoon.

2. Toss in the remaining chickpeas with the parsley, carrot, radishes, and scallions. Stir to combine.

3. In a liquid measuring cup, whisk together the lemon juice, coriander, ½ tsp salt (optional), and fresh ground pepper to taste. Continue whisking while adding the olive oil in a slow stream. Pour over salad and toss gently.

4. Season with salt (optional) and pepper to taste, top with feta and pine nuts (if using), and serve immediately.

Chopped Veggie Tower

This is a salad I've made for years, and I've made many different versions, depending on what I happen to have in my kitchen on any given night. It's a no-brainer, and yet it's so pretty that you can serve it to company. For a Southwestern version, you can add avocado and shredded cheese; or for a Mediterranean version, you can add feta and Greek olives. Let your kids help you choose their favorites and put in the layers—then it's an afternoon art project as well! This recipe serves 8 adult portions.

Ingredients

1 head romaine lettuce, rinsed, dried, and torn into bite-size pieces (about 6 cups loosely packed)

1 cup canned garbanzo beans, drained and rinsed

1 cup canned kidney beans, drained and rinsed

1 cup frozen corn

1 cup canned chopped beets

3 large carrots, chopped

3 stalks celery, chopped

2 medium tomatoes, chopped

1 bunch scallions, chopped

½ cup finely chopped, mixed fresh herbs (e.g. parsley, dill, basil)

½ cup pitted olives, black or green (your choice)

1½ cups low-fat dressing

Option: 2 cups cubed turkey, chicken breast, or ham.

Directions

In a large glass bowl (I use a trifle bowl so you can see all the layers), spread the lettuce on the bottom and layer in the remaining ingredients. Drizzle with dressing before serving.

Corn, Black Bean, and Tomato Salad

This boldly flavored salad is best during spring and summer, when the ingredients are at their peak. Black beans are naturally low in fat and packed with protein, vitamins, and minerals. Plus, they're full of fiber, so they help you feel full. It's an easy way to pack a tasty dish with powerful nutrients and fiber. Serves 4 adult portions.

Ingredients

4–5 ears fresh corn, grilled or boiled and cut off cob

1 can (15-oz) black beans, drained and rinsed

¾ cup grape or plum tomato, chopped

1 T minced red onion, finely chopped

1 T fresh cilantro, chopped

1 jalapeño pepper, seeded and minced (optional)

1 T fresh lime juice

2 tsp olive oil

Salt (optional) and freshly ground pepper to taste

Directions

1.   Combine and mix all of the ingredients in a large bowl, cover, and refrigerate for about 1 hour before serving to allow flavors to blend.

2.   This can be served as a salad (line a bowl with fresh lettuce leaves and spoon in salad), or as a side dish.

Fabulous Fruit Salad

The good thing about a fruit salad is that any combination of fruit will work. Use what's in season and make it look luscious. Keep your fridge full of fruit and offer it in some form at every meal. And if at night your child begs for a peach for dessert instead of ice cream, then you'll know you're doing something right! This recipe should serve 10–12 adult portions.

Ingredients

1 large ripe cantaloupe

1 large ripe honeydew melon

1 pint strawberries cut in half (remove stems)

1 pint blackberries, whole

1 pint raspberries, whole

2 medium bananas, sliced

2 oranges, peeled, seeded, and sectioned

3 ripe peaches, pitted and cut into bite-size pieces

2 cups watermelon rounds or chunks, seeds removed

1 lb seedless grapes cut in half

1 lime

Handful of slivered almonds

Directions

1. Cut melons in half, scoop out seeds, section and peel rind, and cut into bite-size pieces.

2. In a large bowl, combine melon, strawberries, oranges, peaches, and grapes. (Reserve other berries and bananas for later.)

3. Squeeze lime on top and add slivered almonds.

4. Wait till just before serving to toss (I use my hands so as not to bruise fruit). It can be chilled or served at room temperature.

Mozzarella and Tomato Kabobs

I love a Caprese salad, otherwise known as tomato and mozzarella (sometimes it has thinly sliced onions or roasted peppers as well). This version can be served as a salad or as a snack that little ones will find fun to eat. And let's face it, that's the name of the game with kids. If it's enticing, they'll be more likely to try it! And they will get a load of vitamins C and A, calcium, cancer-fighting lycopene, and other protective phytochemicals. This will generally yield 8 adult kabobs, but you can vary the size of the pieces on the kabob according to the age of your child.

Note: Be sure to remove the skewer before serving to children.

Ingredients

1 yellow or red bell pepper, halved and seeded

1 clove garlic, finely chopped

2 T olive oil

1 T fresh lemon juice

16 baby mozzarella balls (Bocaccini)

8 cherry tomatoes, halved

Sea salt (optional) and freshly ground black pepper

16 large fresh basil leaves

8 wood skewers

Directions

1.   Place pepper in oven on broil, cook approximately 8–10 minutes or until charred, then cool and peel. Cut peppers into one-inch squares.

2.   Mix together oil, lemon juice, garlic, and salt (optional) and pepper. Add mozzarella and peppers to marinate 30 minutes.

3.   Thread skewers, first with a cherry tomato half, then a mozzarella ball, then another tomato half, then a pepper square.

4.   Add a basil leaf to each skewer just before serving.

Strawberry, Mango, and Lentil Salad with Balsamic Dressing

This is a mouthwatering combination of flavors, colorful to the eye and packed full of disease-fighting nutrients—beta-carotene, vitamins C and B$_6$, and potassium, as well as fiber and folate. I got this from a friend who knew how much I loved the taste of papaya and mango, and she added that every time she served the dish, she always got rave reviews. I think this is not only a spectacular salad, but also a perfect side dish for chicken, meat, or fish. Serves 4 adult portions.

Ingredients

1 cup lentils

⅓ cup balsamic vinegar

4 tsp olive oil

¾ tsp salt (optional)

½ tsp pepper

1 pint strawberries, quartered

2 cups cherry tomatoes, halved

2 medium mangoes, pitted, peeled, and cut into ½-inch chunks (2 cups)

1 small avocado, pitted, peeled, and cut into ½-inch chunks (¾ cup)

Directions

1. In a large pot of boiling water, cook the lentils until tender but not mushy, about 25 minutes. Then drain.

2. Meanwhile, in a large bowl, whisk together the vinegar, oil, salt, and pepper. Add the warm lentils and toss to combine.

3. Add the strawberries, tomatoes, mangoes, and avocado, and toss again. Serve at room temperature or chilled.

Tomato Salad with Feta, Olives, and Mint

Introducing children to different ethnic cuisines is a big part of the healthy eating adventure. Here's a tasty salad with a Greek flair that will enhance their taste buds . . . and get you out of the kitchen fast!

Ingredients

6 oz feta cheese

¼ cup chopped fresh mint

4 large ripe tomatoes cut into ¼-inch slices

Kosher salt (optional)

½ lb cucumber, peeled, seeded, and diced

½ lb bite-size tomatoes (cherry, pear, or grape) in assorted colors, halved

½ cup Kalamata olives (about 15), pitted and halved

¼ cup extra-virgin olive oil

½ tsp grated lemon zest

4 tsp fresh lemon juice

Freshly ground pepper

Directions

1. Crumble feta into small bowl, add mint, toss, and set aside.

2. Arrange tomato slices, overlapping slightly, on a serving platter.

3. Sprinkle cucumbers over tomato slices.

4. Season the bite-size tomatoes with salt (optional) and scatter them over the cucumber layer. Sprinkle the olives on top.

5. In a small bowl, whisk together the olive oil, lemon zest, and lemon juice. Season to taste with salt (optional) and pepper.

6. To serve, drizzle with vinaigrette and sprinkle remaining feta cheese over salad.

Waldorf Salad with Chicken

I've always loved the combination of flavors in a classic Waldorf, and of course this salad is just filled with fiber and teeming with nutrients. The chicken provides a protein boost and lets it become a meal on its own. It can be served simply on a bed of lettuce, or as we've done here, on cantaloupe, which gives you the added fruit benefit. This recipe serves 4 adult portions.

Ingredients

¼ cup nonfat plain yogurt

¼ cup low-fat mayonnaise

½ tsp honey

1 cup chopped apple (such as McIntosh or Red or Golden Delicious), tossed with 2 tsp fresh lemon juice

½ cup red grapes, halved

½ cup green grapes, halved

½ cup chopped celery

2 T chopped scallions

1 skinless, boneless chicken breast (about 12 oz total), cooked and cubed

1 small cantaloupe, seeds removed and cut into 4 wedges

2 T chopped walnuts, optional

Salt (optional) and pepper to taste

Directions

1. In a large bowl, whisk together the yogurt, mayonnaise, honey, and salt (optional) and pepper to taste.

2. Add the apple, red and green grapes, celery, scallion, and chicken, and toss the mixture well.

3. Mound one-fourth of the salad on top of each wedge of cantaloupe, and top with one-fourth of the walnuts (if using).

19

Soups

Alphabet Soup

Tiny pasta in alphabet shapes makes this soup fun as well as nourishing. It's one of those recipes that can be varied according to what you have in your kitchen on any given day. While Popeye might add a cup of spinach, I've held it to ½ cup in order to make it more appealing to children. It makes eight 1-cup servings.

Ingredients

2 tsp olive oil

1 small onion

1–2 garlic cloves

4 cups tomato juice

1 cup water

1 medium red potato, scrubbed and cut into chunks

1 carrot, cut into chunks

1 stalk celery, sliced

2 tsp Italian herbs

⅛ tsp black pepper

½ cup alphabet pasta

½ cup frozen spinach, thawed and drained

1 15-oz can kidney beans

Directions

1. Heat oil in large pot and add onion and garlic. Cook over medium-high heat until onion is soft, about 5 minutes.

2. Add tomato juice and water, potato, carrot, celery, Italian herbs, and black pepper. Cover and simmer until vegetables are tender, about 20 minutes.

3. Add pasta, chopped spinach, and kidney beans with their liquid. Simmer until spinach and pasta are tender, about 15 minutes. Extra tomato juice or water may be added if thinner soup is desired. Serve.

Butternut Squash Soup

My kids always loved butternut squash and so do I—and it's a good thing, since it's a great source of disease-fighting antioxidants. This delicious soup provides your entire day's requirement of vitamin A and almost a third of your daily vitamin C requirement. Makes 6 adult servings.

Ingredients

1 medium butternut squash (about 2¼ lb)

1 medium onion, chopped (about one cup)

1 T freshly grated ginger (optional)

1 T unsalted butter

3 cups reduced-sodium chicken broth

1 to 2 cups water, or as needed

Salt (optional) and pepper to taste

Low-fat or nonfat sour cream for garnish (optional)

Nonstick vegetable-oil spray

Directions

1. Preheat oven to 400°F.

2. Cut squash in half lengthwise, and scoop out and discard seeds.

3. Arrange the halves, cut side down, in roasting pan that has been sprayed with nonstick vegetable-oil spray. Bake squash for 40 to 45 minutes, or until tender. Set aside to cool.

4. When squash is completely cooked, scoop out flesh.

5. While squash is baking, melt butter in saucepan and cook onion and ginger over moderately low heat for 5 minutes or until onion is softened.

6. Add onion mixture to squash pulp and transfer to blender or food processor, in batches. Puree until smooth. Add enough water to get desired consistency. Add salt (optional) and pepper to taste.

7. Return pureed mixture to saucepan. Add broth and simmer covered for 10 minutes.

8. Garnish with dollop of sour cream.

9. Serve in hollowed-out baby pumpkin halves to really delight your family.

Old-Fashioned Chicken Soup

You know the theory that chicken soup is the best cure-all for whatever ails you? Well the best thing actually is that you don't have to be sick to enjoy it! When Dr. Winick spoke to me about the value of using bones in soup recipes to increase the intake of calcium, I immediately thought of this one. It makes 10 to 12 adult servings.

Ingredients

1 package marrow or soup bones (about 4 bones)

1 3½-lb chicken (preferably kosher), rinsed and cut up

1 large onion, cut into eighths

2 large carrots, halved

1 stalk celery, halved

2 large parsnips, halved

1 small bunch dill

1 small bunch parsley

Salt (optional) and pepper to taste

Optional: cooked white rice, soup noodles or matzo balls (prepared according to package directions)

Directions

1. In a large pot, combine soup bones, chicken, and enough water to cover by two inches. Bring water to boil and simmer 20 minutes, skimming as needed.

2. Add vegetables, dill, and parsley (I always bunch the herbs together with a rubber band around them so I can remove them later), and bring soup back to a boil. Simmer for 2 hours.

3. Skim fat, strain stock and remove chicken from the bones (discard all bones) and herb bouquet.

4. In a clean pot, combine strained stock with chicken meat, and add the sliced vegetables. Season to taste with salt (optional) and pepper.

5. Cook soup over medium-high heat until hot and ladle over rice, noodles, or matzo balls, if desired.

Sweet Corn Chowder

Little kids usually like the sweet taste of corn and it's a wonderful source of fiber, which may inhibit the growth of cancer cells. I recommend you make the crab cakes on page 260 with this soup recipe. Then ladle 6 to 8 ounces of the soup into individual bowls and place crab cake on top. Serves 6 adult portions.

Ingredients

4 cups fresh corn kernels (or frozen corn)

3 T corn oil

1 medium onion, peeled and chopped (about ½ cup)

1 jalapeño pepper, stem and seeds removed, chopped roughly

1 clove fresh garlic, peeled and sliced

1¾ tsp ground coriander

3½ to 4 cups skim milk

1 tsp kosher salt (optional)

½ tsp freshly ground black pepper

Directions

1. Heat corn oil in a large saucepan. Sauté onion, pepper, and garlic over medium heat for about 5 minutes or until soft. Add the ground coriander and stir for about 30 seconds. Add corn kernels, salt (optional), pepper, and milk. Bring to boil and cook at a simmer, covered, about 40 minutes. Stir occasionally.

2. Remove from heat and place 1½ cups of hot soup in blender. Place cover on blender and hold firmly in place while blending. Blend until smooth. Place blended portion in a clean saucepan and blend remaining soup in 1½-cup batches. Taste for seasoning and adjust with salt (optional) and pepper as needed. Serve.

Cucumber-Yogurt Soup with Avocado

This is a no-cook soup that's quick to make in the food processor. Simply chill and serve cold. As the soup chills, the flavors meld and the texture becomes smoother. This soup contains calcium and phytonutrients, which protect against disease. This recipe makes about six cups.

Ingredients

1 large white onion, preferably sweet (8-oz), quartered

1 lb cucumbers, peeled, seeded and cut into big chunks

1 medium-size ripe avocado

1½ cups plain yogurt

3 T extra-virgin olive oil

1 clove garlic, minced

¾ tsp ground cumin (toasted and freshly ground if available)

1 tsp kosher salt (optional)

⅓ cup loosely packed fresh basil leaves

2 T fresh mint leaves

2–3 T fresh lemon juice

Freshly ground black pepper

Directions

1. Place onion in food processor; pulse to chop finely, place in colander, rinse under cold water and set aside to drain.

2. Place cucumber chunks in processor; pulse to chop finely. Add back the drained onion and pulse to combine. Set aside ¾ cup of cucumber-onion mix to stir into soup at end.

3. Cut avocado in half; remove pit, scoop out pulp and place in processor with remaining cucumber-onion mix. Add yogurt, olive oil, garlic, cumin, and salt (optional). Puree until smooth and transfer to bowl.

4. Slice basil and mint leaves into shreds with sharp knife. Stir into soup along with lemon juice, 1 cup cold water, and reserved cucumber-onion mixture.

5. Season to taste with salt (optional) and pepper. Cover and chill for several hours.

6. Before serving, check consistency and if necessary, add another ½ to 1 cup cold water (you may also want to add more lemon juice and salt).

7. Garnish with a few shredded mint leaves and serve.

Lentils and Seashell Soup

This recipe comes from Lisa Vitiello, who has a wonderful Italian restaurant in Greenwich, Connecticut, which my family loves. Lisa says this kind of ordinary peasant food was a staple when she was growing up on the island of Ischia on the Amalfi Coast in southern Italy. She says all of her grandchildren adore it—Anthony, thirteen, Victoria, ten, Ariana, four, Joey, five, and even little Johnny, who is only one year old. It's teeming with nutritious ingredients, yet it's very easy to make.

Ingredients

8 oz sorted lentils

1 carrot finely chopped

1 small diced onion

1 small diced potato

1 clove finely chopped garlic

½ cup extra-virgin olive oil

3 fresh or canned plum tomatoes (optional)

4 oz small pasta shells

3 fresh basil leaves (optional)

Directions

1. Sort and rinse lentils. Place in a pan with cold water and bring to boil.

2. Add olive oil, onion, garlic, tomatoes, carrots, and potatoes. Let all ingredients simmer for about 35 to 45 minutes, stirring occasionally.

3. Add chopped basil when lentils are fully cooked for wonderful flavor and aroma.

4. Small amounts of water may be added while cooking, as needed, if lentil soup appears too dry.

5. In a separate pan, bring cold water to boil and add shells. Cook until done, drain thoroughly and add to lentils. Serve.

Minestrone

This is classic minestrone from the renowned Patsy's Italian restaurant in New York City. The beauty of this basic recipe is that you can use all the vegetables (packed full of powerful vitamins and protective nutrients!) or just those you happen to have in your kitchen at the time. There's no one right way to make minestrone. This recipe serves 16 to 18 adult portions, and I recommend cooking up a pot so that you can get several meals for those days when you just don't have time.

Ingredients

½ cup olive oil

2 medium yellow onions, finely chopped

3 celery ribs, trimmed and finely chopped

3–4 garlic cloves, minced

1 28-oz can plum tomatoes, with juice

2 medium carrots, diced

2 medium Idaho potatoes, peeled and cubed

1 medium cauliflower (about 2 lbs) separated into florets

2 medium zucchini, cubed

1 10-oz package frozen peas, thawed

1 15-oz can cannellini beans, rinsed and drained

¾ lb orzo pasta, cooked al dente

3 T chopped fresh parsley

3 T basil

Salt (optional) and freshly ground pepper to taste

Directions

1. Heat oil in a large soup pot over medium-high heat and sauté onion and celery for 6 to 7 minutes, or until lightly browned. Reduce heat to low and sauté garlic until golden, about 1 to 2 minutes.

2. Coarsely chop the tomatoes and add to pot with their juice. Increase the heat to high and add carrots, potatoes, cauliflower, and 12 cups water. Bring pot to a boil, reduce heat to low, cover, and simmer for 15 to 18 minutes.

3. Add zucchini, peas, and beans, and bring to a boil again. Reduce heat to low, cover, and simmer for additional 15–18 minutes.

4. Add cooked pasta, basil, and parsley. Season with salt (optional) and pepper to taste, and simmer for an additional 2 minutes, or until pasta is heated through. Serve.

Pasta e Fagioli Soup

This classic Italian soup, which combines pasta and beans, has always been a favorite with my girls. The recipe comes from our friends at Patsy's Italian restaurant in New York City. It's loaded with nutrients but doesn't take a load of work to prepare. Serves 6 adult portions.

Ingredients

¼ cup olive oil

1 yellow onion, diced

2 celery ribs, trimmed and chopped

2 small carrots, chopped

2 cloves garlic, minced

1 14-oz can plum tomatoes, with juice

6 cups vegetable broth

1 15-oz can cannellini beans, rinsed and drained

½ lb ziti pasta, cooked al dente

Salt (optional) and freshly ground pepper to taste

⅓ cup fresh parsley

Directions

1. Heat the oil in a large saucepan over medium-high flame and sauté the onion, celery, and carrot, stirring occasionally, for 3 minutes or until onions are just translucent. Add the garlic and sauté 1 minute or until lightly golden.

2. Coarsely chop the tomatoes and add with their juice to the saucepan. Add the broth and bring to a boil. Cover, reduce heat to low, and simmer for 20 minutes.

3. Add cannellini beans and cooked pasta, stir to combine, and simmer for an additional 5–6 minutes, or until all ingredients are heated through. Season with salt (optional) and pepper to taste.

4. Stir in parsley and simmer for 2 more minutes. Serve.

Pastina à la Patsy's

first took my daughters, Jamie, Lindsay, and Sarah, to Patsy's Italian restaurant in New York City when they were only toddlers and needed booster seats. While other patrons enjoyed classic gourmet dishes like Osso Bucco and Cannelloni, my little ones made a meal of pastina and warm garlic bread. It's a good bet that your children will love this simple dish as well. And you'll love how easy it is to prepare. Serves 4 adult portions.

Ingredients

½ lb chicken wings and bones

8 cups cold water

1 8-oz can plum tomatoes

2 onions, quartered

3 carrots cut into 2-inch pieces

4 celery ribs trimmed and quartered

3 bay leaves

4 crushed peppercorns

Salt to taste (optional)

1½ cups pastina

Directions

1. Rinse the chicken parts and put them in a large soup pot. Add cold water and remaining ingredients, except salt and pastina. Bring to a boil, reduce heat, and simmer. Some foam will form from the chicken bones. With a slotted spoon, skim foam off. You may have to do this more than once.

2. Simmer for 3 to 4 hours. Add salt to taste (optional).

3. Pass through a very fine strainer and return to heat. Bring back to boil and add pastina. Simmer 4 to 5 minutes. Serve.

Sweet Potato Soup

This is so sweet your kids will love it, and it's so easy that you'll love it. And it's filled with beta-carotene, so their growing bodies will love it, too! Recipe serves 6 adult portions.

Ingredients

1 T vegetable oil

1 small onion, chopped

6 cups reduced-sodium chicken stock

2 large sweet potatoes, peeled and chopped

½ tsp ground nutmeg

¼ tsp freshly ground pepper

Directions

1. In a large saucepan, warm oil over medium-high heat. Add onion and sauté for 2–3 minutes or until onion is soft and translucent. Add chicken stock, sweet potatoes, nutmeg, and pepper. Cover and bring to a boil; reduce heat and simmer for 25 minutes or until potatoes are tender.

2. Remove soup from heat, and in batches, puree soup in a blender or food processor until smooth. Return soup to saucepan and heat thoroughly.

3. Garnish soup with dollop of nonfat sour cream or yogurt. Serve.

Tortilla Soup

While I was in college, I studied for several years in Mexico, and while I was there I will confess I fell in love. That's right, I fell in love with tortilla soup. This recipe reminds me of the kind I found south of the border, hot and spicy! Makes about 7 adult servings.

Ingredients

1 medium onion, chopped (about 1 cup)

2 garlic cloves, minced (about 2 tsp)

2 T vegetable oil

4-oz can green chilies, chopped

15-oz can Italian-style stewed tomatoes, chopped, reserving the juice

4 cups fresh chicken broth or canned reduced-sodium chicken broth

1 tsp lemon pepper

2 tsp Worcestershire sauce

1 tsp chili powder

1 tsp ground cumin

½ tsp hot sauce or to taste

4 T all-purpose flour

½ cup water

1 lb skinless boneless chicken breast, cut into small cubes

⅓ cup nonfat or low-fat sour cream

Salt (optional) and pepper to taste

Tortilla strips (recipe follows)

Chopped fresh coriander for garnish (optional)

Directions

1. In a large saucepan, cook onion and garlic in oil over moderately low heat for 5 minutes or until onion is softened.

2. Add the chilies, tomatoes with their juice, broth, lemon pepper, Worcestershire, spices, and hot sauce and simmer the mixture for 20 minutes.

3. In a small bowl, combine the flour with the water and whisk it into the soup. Bring the soup back to a boil and simmer for 5 minutes.

4. Add the chicken and simmer for 5 minutes or until it is just cooked through.

5. Stir in the sour cream and salt (optional) and pepper to taste, and garnish each portion with tortilla strips (recipe below) and coriander, if desired.

Tortilla Strips

Ingredients

> **4 corn tortillas cut into ¼-inch strips**
>
> **Nonstick vegetable-oil spray**

Directions

Preheat the oven to 400°F.

1. Arrange the tortilla strips in one layer in a baking pan sprayed with vegetable oil.

2. Bake 10 minutes or until lightly toasted and crispy.

3. Sprinkle lightly with salt, if desired.

20

Meatless Main Dishes and Pastas

Eggplant Parmesan

Eggplants are high in fiber and low in fat, and they have a "meaty" texture that makes them ideal for this sumptuous recipe. Of course I always thought that "eggplant parmesan" was fattening, but this version lets us enjoy all the flavors of the classic dish, without the fat.

Ingredients

2 small eggplants (about 2 lb total)

Nonstick vegetable-oil spray

Juice of 1 lemon

Salt (optional) and pepper to taste

1½ cups roasted fresh tomato sauce or your favorite purchased brand

4 oz low-fat mozzarella, coarsely grated

¼ cup chopped parsley

⅓ cup freshly grated Parmesan (about 2½ oz)

Directions

1. Preheat the oven to 400°F.

2. Peel the eggplants and slice them crosswise ½-inch thick.

3. Arrange the slices in one layer on a baking sheet sprayed with the nonstick vegetable-oil spray, and sprinkle them with the lemon juice and salt (optional) and pepper to taste.

(continued)

4. Bake for 10 minutes; turn them over and bake for an additional 10 minutes or until golden.

5. Spread 2 tablespoons of the tomato sauce in the bottom of an 8-inch round quiche pan or pie plate.

6. Arrange one-half of the eggplant slices over the sauce, overlapping them slightly, and top the eggplant with half of the remaining tomato sauce, half of the mozzarella, half of the parsley, and half of the Parmesan.

7. Repeat the procedure with the remaining ingredients, and bake for 30 minutes or until very hot and bubbly.

(The Eggplant Parmesan can be made ahead and reheated at 350°F for 30–40 minutes.)

Vegetable Lasagna

Most kids love lasagna, and it's an easy way to add veggies and lots of calcium. I looked for an easy recipe that didn't take too long. This one really fits the bill. Since you don't precook the noodles your prep time is cut in half, and it's easy to include lots of green veggies amidst the layers of noodles! This recipe makes about 12 adult servings. If you don't eat it all at one sitting, it's great the next day and freezes well.

Ingredients

15-oz container low-fat ricotta cheese

1 cup low-fat cottage cheese (or mashed firm tofu)

1 tsp chopped garlic

½ tsp dried basil

½ tsp freshly grated Parmesan cheese

4 cups spaghetti sauce

12 lasagna noodles (¾ lb)

2 cups (8 oz) grated part-skim mozzarella cheese

1¼ cups steamed chopped broccoli or chopped spinach

Directions

1. Preheat oven to 350°F.

2. Spray 9-by-13-inch pan with vegetable-oil cooking spray.

3. Mix together ricotta, cottage cheese, basil, and Parmesan.

4. Assemble ingredients in this order: 1 cup sauce on bottom of pan, 4 noodles touching, ½ of cheese mixture, ⅔ cup mozzarella, ⅓ of veggies. Repeat until all ingredients are used, finishing with one layer of pasta, topped with sauce and mozzarella.

5. Cover pan tightly with tin foil and bake 1 to 1½ hours (depending on your oven). Serve.

Savory Black Beans and Rice

Dr. Winick often suggests this dish as a perfect protein substitute for those who don't eat meat. My brother Jeff began cooking this recipe when he was in the navy stationed in Puerto Rico. It's one of those dishes you can serve as a main course, as an accompaniment to fajitas or burritos, or as a side dish to grilled meat or poultry. Try using salsa for an added kick. Serves 6 adult portions.

Ingredients

2 cups reduced-sodium chicken broth

1 cup long-grain rice

1 medium onion, chopped finely (about 1 cup)

2 garlic cloves, minced (about 2 tsp)

2 tsp olive oil

2 16-oz cans black beans, drained and rinsed

1 cup canned crushed tomatoes or 1 cup salsa, mild or medium

2 T red wine vinegar

¼ tsp cayenne pepper, or to taste

2–3 T chopped fresh cilantro, or to taste

Salt and pepper to taste

Directions

1. In a saucepan, combine the chicken broth and rice and bring to a boil. Reduce heat to low, cover tightly, and simmer for 18 to 20 minutes, or until the rice is tender and all liquid has been absorbed.

2. While rice is cooking, in a large nonstick skillet cook the onion and garlic in oil over moderate heat for 5 minutes, or until onion is softened. Add the beans, tomatoes or salsa, vinegar, and cayenne, and simmer for 5 minutes.

3. Stir in reserved rice, cilantro, and salt and pepper to taste.

Vegetable Fajitas

Mexican food of any kind is always a favorite around my house, and fajitas are especially easy to make. It's one of those "no-brainer" quick dinners. This recipe calls for lots of health-promoting vegetables and is a colorful dish. Serves 4 adult portions.

Ingredients

8 flour or whole-wheat tortillas (8-inch diameter)

2 T vegetable oil

1 small onion, peeled and cut into thin strips

1 small red bell pepper, seeded and sliced thinly

1 small green bell pepper, seeded and sliced thinly

1 tsp minced garlic

1 medium yellow summer squash, cut into 2-inch strips

1 cup salsa or picante sauce

1 tsp ground cumin

½ tsp salt (optional)

1 cup shredded Monterey Jack cheese (low-fat)

¼ cup chopped fresh cilantro (optional)

Directions

1. Wrap tortillas in aluminum foil and place in 350°F oven for 15 minutes, or until thoroughly heated.

2. In a 10-inch skillet, heat oil over medium-high heat. Cook onion, red and green peppers, and garlic, stir to cover with oil. Cover, reduce heat to medium, and cook for 5 minutes. Stir squash into vegetables; then stir in salsa, cumin, and salt. Cover and cook for 5 minutes.

3. Spoon vegetable mixture evenly down the center of the warm tortillas and sprinkle with cheese and cilantro. Roll up the tortillas and serve.

Emilio's Mac 'n' Cheese Italian Style

If kids came with little instruction manuals, I'm sure they would say somewhere, "When hungry, just feed macaroni and cheese." Come on, have you ever heard of a little child not liking macaroni and cheese? So here's a new twist on an old favorite from Sergio Brasesco, a wonderful chef and owner of Emilio's in Harrison, New York. This recipe serves 4 adult portions.

Ingredients

1 box fusilli pasta (multicolored if possible)

½ cup low-fat Alpine Lace Swiss cheese (buy it in a chunk, not sliced)

1 tsp sweet unsalted butter

½ cup Grana Padano cheese, grated

Splash of olive oil

Directions

1. Cut Alpine Lace Swiss into sugar-cube-sized pieces. Set aside. (If Alpine Lace Swiss is not available, you can use any cheese you desire.)

2. Boil pasta in salted water, according to package directions.

3. Once pasta is ready, drain, splash with olive oil, and return to pot.

4. Add butter and cubed Alpine Lace cheese. Cover pot and shake it up! Allow cheese to melt and coat the pasta.

5. Put onto plates, sprinkle Grana Padano cheese on top, and serve.

Fettuccini Tossed with Fresh Tomatoes and Basil

The famous Italian restaurant Patsy's in New York City is one of my favorites. Besides the warm and friendly atmosphere, it has exquisite food. I asked them to share with you a recipe for fettuccini that tastes "oh so fresh," because you can make it at the last minute, with just a little preparation earlier in the afternoon. This recipe serves 6 adult portions.

Ingredients

3 large ripe tomatoes, diced (about 4 cups)

½ cup (loosely packed) shredded fresh basil leaves

6–8 garlic cloves, thinly sliced, to taste

⅓ cup plus 2 T extra-virgin olive oil

Salt (optional) and freshly ground black pepper, to taste

1 lb fettuccine, cooked al dente

1 cup grated provolone (about 4 oz)

Directions

1. In a large bowl, combine the tomatoes, basil, garlic, and ⅓ cup of oil. Season to taste with salt (optional) and pepper. Cover and marinate at room temperature for 3 hours.

2. Add cooked fettuccini to the tomato mixture, sprinkle with cheese and remaining oil, and toss. Serve.

Pumpkin and Sage Risotto with Mushroom and Pea Ragout

Risotto gets its creamy consistency from the arborio rice, its main ingredient. You can add meat, seafood, mushrooms, and just about any kind of vegetable to the dish. Risotto requires more of your time and attention in the kitchen, so this is not an everyday dish—but I think you'll agree that the results are worth the effort. I'm especially fond of this recipe, which uses pumpkin, a potent immunity booster and cancer fighter. Topped with the Mushroom and Pea Ragout, from our friends at the *Good Housekeeping* test kitchen; it's not only delicious it's a complete protein. Serves 6 to 8 adult portions.

Ingredients

Risotto

6 cups reduced-sodium chicken broth

½ cup canned pumpkin

1 small onion, finely chopped

1 T olive oil

3 cups cubed, peeled pumpkin or butternut squash

2 cups arborio rice

⅓ cup dry white wine or reduced-sodium chicken broth

½ cup grated Parmesan cheese

2 tsp fresh sage

Ground pepper

Mushroom and Pea Ragout

1 T olive oil

1 small onion or shallot, chopped

1 small garlic clove, crushed

2 packages mixed exotic mushrooms (8 oz total)

1 box (10 oz) frozen peas, thawed

¼ cup reduced-sodium chicken broth

Directions

Risotto

1. In a large saucepan, stir together broth and canned pumpkin. Bring to a boil. Reduce heat and simmer.

2. Meanwhile, in a 4-quart Dutch oven, cook onion in hot oil over medium heat for about 5 minutes or until tender. Add fresh pumpkin or squash and cook for 2 minutes, stirring. Add in uncooked rice, stirring for two more minutes.

3. Slowly add wine to the rice mixture and cook until the wine is evaporated. Slowly add 2 cups of the broth mixture, stirring constantly. Continue to cook and stir until liquid is absorbed. Add the remaining broth mixture, ¾ cup at a time, stirring constantly until the broth is absorbed (about 30 minutes).

4. Stir the Parmesan cheese and sage into rice mixture. Season to taste with black pepper. You can serve this with or over a green vegetable like broccoli or spinach.

Ragout

1. Sauté onion in 10-inch skillet over medium heat until tender and golden, about 10 minutes. Add garlic and cook 30 seconds.

2. Stir in mushrooms; increase heat to medium-high, and cook 5 minutes until mushrooms are wilted.

3. Stir in peas and broth and cook until heated through.

4. Serve about ½ cup portion in the center of each bowl of risotto.

Gail's Brown Rice Casserole

This recipe comes to us compliments of Gail North, one of the writers who worked diligently researching and assembling all of the facts in this book to help us as parents know what to feed our children so that we can give them the best protection against disease. Brown rice is, of course, packed with protection as well as vitamins and fiber. It took a little effort and cajoling at first to get my family to make the switch from white rice to brown rice, but now we like to keep brown rice in the fridge at all times. By the way, if you're pressed for time, use canned beans. You can add other veggies, or pieces of cooked chicken—be creative, and you'll easily get a second meal out of this dish. This recipe serves 4–6 adult portions.

Ingredients

2 cups short-grain brown rice

3 T tamari or soy sauce (low-sodium)

2 bunches scallions, chopped finely with green parts

½ cup fresh dill (packed), chopped coarsely

½ cup fresh Italian parsley (packed), chopped coarsely

1 cup steamed broccoli florets

½ cup fresh or frozen peas

1 cup cooked black beans (or red beans) (fresh or canned)

Dash freshly ground pepper

½ cup tahini sauce (sesame sauce)

½ cup chopped almonds (optional)

Directions

1. Cook brown rice according to directions (2 cups rice to 4 cups water).

2. After rice is cooked, add tamari or soy sauce and mix.

3. Toss in chopped scallions, dill, parsley, broccoli florets, and peas, and mix.

4. Add black or red beans and pepper and mix again.

5. Drizzle tahini sauce into rice. Mix well.

6. Mix in chopped almonds, if desired.

7. Transfer rice to a serving bowl, garnish with parsley leaves, and serve.

This dish can be served hot or cold. Try it both ways.

Garden Pizza

asked my friends at the *Good Housekeeping* test kitchen for an easy vegetable pizza, and they crafted this delicious, nutrient-rich pizza that should delight you and your kids. You can make the dough yourself or you can substitute refrigerated or frozen dough. I think it's a good idea to keep some refrigerated dough on hand for those last-minute pizza cravings. Serves 8 adult portions.

Ingredients

Topping

1 T vegetable oil

1 small zucchini (6 oz), cut into ¼-inch pieces

1 small yellow straight neck squash (6 oz), cut into ¼-inch pieces

1 large tomato, seeded and cut into ¼-inch pieces

½ tsp dried oregano

¼ tsp ground black pepper

¼ tsp salt (optional)

1 cup shredded part-skim mozzarella cheese

Directions

1. Prepare Quick Homemade Pizza Dough (see next page), or use refrigerated pizza dough.

2. Preheat oven to 450°F.

3. In a 12-inch skillet, heat oil over medium-high heat. Add zucchini and yellow squash and cook until tender. Stir in tomato, oregano, pepper, and salt (optional).

4. Top pizza dough with squash mixture. Sprinkle evenly with shredded mozzarella cheese.

5. Bake pizza on bottom rack of oven until crust is golden and crisp, 20 to 25 minutes.

6. Cut into wedges and serve.

Quick Homemade Pizza Dough

Ingredients

2½ cups all-purpose flour

1 package quick-rise yeast

1 tsp salt (optional)

1 cup very warm water (120 to 130°F)

2 tsp cornmeal

Directions

1. In a large bowl, combine 2 cups flour, yeast, and salt (optional). Stir in very warm water until blended and dough comes away from the sides of the bowl.

2. Turn dough onto floured surface and knead until smooth and elastic, about 8 minutes, working in more flour (the remaining ½ cup) while kneading. Shape dough into a ball, cover with plastic wrap, and let rest 10 minutes.

3. Grease a 15-inch pizza pan and sprinkle with cornmeal. Pat dough onto bottom of pizza pan, shaping dough into ½-inch-high rim at edge of pan.

Option: Substitute 1 package (10 oz) refrigerated pizza dough and press into 15-inch pizza pan as directed in step 3 above.

21

Chicken and Beef

Baked "Baby" Meatballs

Lisa Vitiello takes pleasure cooking for her patrons at Da Vinci's Italian restaurant in Greenwich, Connecticut, but she also loves cooking for her grandchildren, and this one is always a crowd-pleaser. She especially likes this recipe because it's so versatile. The meatballs can be served alone (she says her kids always liked them warm out of the oven), or with pasta and a quick tomato sauce. For older children, she suggests serving them on a roll or preferably on whole wheat bread as a nutritious and hearty sandwich.

Meatballs

Ingredients

1 lb extra lean chopped meat

1 egg

¼ cup chopped Italian parsley

2 cloves chopped garlic

2 T imported Parmesan cheese

¼ tsp oregano

½ cup bread crumbs

Directions

1. Mix all ingredients well in a mixing bowl and form into small meatballs (little kids like the smaller size).

2. Place on baking pan with a little water. Bake at 400°F for approximately 25 to 30 minutes.

Quick Tomato Sauce

Ingredients

25-oz can Italian plum tomatoes, strained

½ cup extra-virgin olive oil

1 medium-size onion, chopped

1 clove garlic chopped

6 fresh chopped basil leaves

2 T chopped Italian parsley

Directions

1. Sauté onion and garlic in olive oil until brown. Add tomatoes and simmer for approximately 25 minutes.

2. Stir in chopped basil and parsley. Adding these herbs after the cooking process is over enhances their wonderful fresh aromas that might otherwise be lost if added too early on in the cooking process.

Chicken and Barley

My mom always told me that even if she got home late in the afternoon, she would throw a few onions in a pan and get them cooking . . . and when my dad walked in it smelled like she had been cooking all day! This dish will make your house smell incredibly good. It's chocked full of nutrients and flavor and your kids will love it too. Serves four.

Ingredients

Vegetable-oil spray

1½ lbs of chicken parts, patted dry and seasoned with salt and pepper (you can use leg, thigh, or breast, skin removed)

¼ lb sweet Italian sausage, casing removed and chopped

1 small onion, chopped

1 red pepper, seeded and diced

1–2 cloves garlic, finely chopped

2 cups pearl barley

1 tsp ground cumin

½ teaspoon chili powder

1 bay leaf

14½-oz can peeled, crushed tomatoes

2½ cups water

Directions

1. In a heavy soup pan or Dutch oven, sauté sausage in oil for 3 minutes or until brown. Remove to platter. Add chicken and cook for 10 minutes, turning pieces often, until golden on all sides. Remove chicken, set aside, and drain oil from pan.

2. Lightly spray pan with vegetable oil again, and sauté the onion, pepper, and garlic for about 2 minutes. Stir in the barley, add the seasonings, the tomatoes, and water. Bring to a boil, cover, and reduce the heat to a simmer. Cook for 20 minutes. Add more water if needed.

3. Add the chicken and sausage back into pot and cook an additional 25 to 30 minutes until chicken is completely cooked and barley is tender. Add another ½ cup water if barley looks dry.

Baked *Fried* Chicken

Whoever figured out how to make fried chicken without frying it should get some kind of major award, don't you think? Really, to take the fat out of one of the most fattening meals, one that's practically a signature dish here in the good ole USA, is downright patriotic, if you ask me. Whether out at a picnic or at home, you can't lose with this one from *Good Housekeeping* magazine! Serves 4 adult portions.

Ingredients

½ cup plain dried bread crumbs

¼ cup freshly grated Parmesan cheese

2 T cornmeal

½ tsp ground cayenne pepper

1 large egg white

½ tsp salt

1 chicken (3½ lb), cut into 8 pieces and skin removed from all but wings

Nonstick olive-oil cooking spray

Directions

1. Preheat the oven to 425°F. Grease 15½-by-10½ jelly roll pan with cooking spray.

2. On waxed paper, combine bread crumbs, Parmesan cheese, cornmeal, and cayenne pepper. In a pie plate, beat egg white and salt.

3. Dip each piece of chicken in egg-white mixture, then coat with crumb mixture, firmly pressing so mixture adheres. Arrange chicken in prepared pan; lightly coat chicken with cooking spray.

4. Bake chicken until coating is crisp and golden brown and juices run clear when thickest part of chicken is pierced with tip of knife, about 35 minutes.

Chicken Enchiladas

Mexican dishes usually go over big with my kids, and these enchiladas are delicious and nutritious. This recipe is a favorite of Tammie Sanchez, a trained chef who has cooked for the young children at my husband's summer camps for several years. I suggest you serve them with Mexican rice and my Chunky Guacamole Salad. This makes about 8 enchiladas, depending on how you stuff them.

Ingredients

4 skinless boneless chicken breasts

2 (10-oz) cans of Old El Paso enchilada sauce

6 oz (about 1½ cup) shredded light cheddar cheese

1 package light wheat flour tortillas

1 T chopped cilantro

1 T minced garlic

¼ cup chopped green onion

1 jalapeño, chopped fine

1 can (about ¼ cup) Old El Paso green chilies

Salt (optional) and pepper to taste

Directions

1. Bake chicken at 350°F until cooked through. Squeeze a little lemon juice on chicken along with a dash of salt (optional) and pepper. (A little garlic is optional.) When finished baking, shred meat and set aside.

2. Combine chicken, 1 can of enchilada sauce, 1 cup cheese, cilantro, minced garlic, green onion, jalapeño pepper, green chilies, salt (optional) and pepper, and stir.

3. Spoon filling inside tortillas, roll up and place in a 13 x 9 x 2-inch baking dish.

4. Pour the remaining enchilada sauce over the top. Sprinkle on the remaining cheese (½ cup), and a small handful of green onions. Bake at 375°F for 15–20 minutes.

Chicken and Corn Chilaquiles Casserole

My daughter Lindsay loves to cook, so she worked a summer internship in the testing kitchens of *Good Housekeeping* magazine. She felt that it was a dream job, cooking and eating scrumptious dishes. And she thought that this casserole recipe, which got the food department's Seal of Approval, would delight your kids and not keep you in the kitchen for too long. It makes 4 main-dish adult servings

Ingredients

3 cups baked, unsalted tortilla chips

1 jar (14 oz) verde sauce with tomatillos and jalapeño chilies

2 packages (4 oz each) roasted chicken breast halves; skin removed and meat pulled into shreds

1 package (10 oz) frozen corn kernels

½ 8-oz package shredded low-fat Monterey Jack or Mexican cheese blend (1 cup)

¼ cup loosely packed fresh cilantro leaves, chopped (optional)

Directions

1. Preheat oven to 375°F. In deep 2½-quart ceramic or glass baking dish, spread half of the chips, overlapping slightly. Top with half of the sauce, chicken, corn, and cheese. Repeat layers.

2. Cover dish with glass lid or nonstick foil. Bake covered for 20 minutes. Remove lid and bake 5 to 10 minutes longer, or until cheese melts.

3. Sprinkle with cilantro and serve.

Penne with Chicken and Broccoli

Okay, let's all agree—pasta is the universal food among kids. So, it's the perfect dish for sneaking in a little protein and some vegetables teeming with nutrients and fiber. This recipe, from Lisa Vitiello of Da Vinci's restaurant in Greenwich, Connecticut, is fairly quick and easy, and provides children with their vegetable, protein, and carbs in a tasty, satisfying dish. Serves 8 to 10.

Ingredients

1 lb penne

½ cup extra-virgin olive oil

3 cloves garlic

2 boneless, skinless, and cubed chicken breasts

2 cups broccoli florets, thoroughly cleaned

8 oz low-sodium chicken broth

Directions

1. Boil pasta approximately 10 minutes or to desired consistency and taste.

2. Sauté garlic in olive oil until golden.

3. Add the cubed chicken and continue sautéing until chicken loses its pink color.

4. Remove the chicken from the pan and place on the side.

5. Add broccoli florets and sauté—add chicken broth, cover pan with lid so as to allow thorough cooking of broccoli.

6. Add penne and chicken to broth mixture.

7. Serve with a sprinkle of Parmesan cheese if desired.

Penne with Fresh Peas and Prosciutto

From Wolfgang Puck's
Pizza, Pasta, and More!

learned a lot about cooking from Wolfgang Puck, who was a regular visitor to our set at *Good Morning America*. This recipe from his book *Pizza, Pasta, and More!* should be a kid pleaser. Wolfgang says if the ingredients are readied early in the day, you can make the sauce while the pasta is cooking and have this dish on the table as soon as the pasta is al dente. Serves 4 to 6 adult portions.

Ingredients

3 T extra-virgin olive oil

½ medium white onion (about 4 oz), peeled and chopped finely

2 T pulp of whole roasted garlic

1½ cups chicken stock (heated)

¼ cup freshly grated Parmesan cheese, plus more for garnish

3 oz goat cheese, crumbled

4 T (½ stick) unsalted butter, cut into small pieces

½ tsp fresh oregano leaves, minced

½ tsp fresh thyme leaves, minced

Kosher salt (optional) and freshly ground white pepper

12 oz penne (or tubular pasta of your choice)

2 cups shelled fresh peas (about ½ lb), blanched

½ cup oven-dried tomatoes cut into strips (or sun-dried tomatoes)

¼ lb prosciutto, cut into thin strips

Chopped fresh flat leaf parsley leaves for garnish

Directions

1. Fill a large stockpot with water and bring it to a boil.

2. In a large sauté pan, heat olive oil over medium heat and sauté onion until golden. Add garlic, pour in stock, and stir in Parmesan cheese, goat cheese, and butter. Cook just until the sauce thickens slightly. Season with oregano, thyme, and salt (optional) and pepper to taste.

3. Meanwhile, cook the penne until al dente and drain. Add the penne to the sauce and stir to coat well. Stir in the peas and tomatoes, and cook for 1 to 2 minutes longer. Just before you are ready to serve, stir in the prosciutto and adjust the seasonings to taste.

4. To serve, divide the pasta among 4 heated plates or bowls, making certain that you spoon some of the peas, tomatoes, prosciutto, and sauce over each serving. Garnish with chopped parsley and grated Parmesan cheese, if desired.

To prepare ahead: Have all the ingredients ready, including the blanched peas, and continue with the recipe when ready to serve.

Linguini with Chicken Bolognese

From Wolfgang Puck's
Pizza, Pasta, and More!

This Chicken Bolognese makes a nourishing low-fat pasta sauce. And it freezes well so you can have it at a moment's notice. I suggest making a big batch on a quiet Sunday afternoon and freezing in dinner-size containers for those hectic "after-school" afternoons when you just can't deal with carpools, homework, baths, and dinner preparation. Wolfgang adds that the vegetables can be cut as described below, giving the sauce texture, or if you prefer, they can be pureed in a blender or food processor for a smoother sauce. Makes about 5½ adult servings.

Ingredients

5 T olive oil

2 lb coarsely ground chicken, preferably dark meat

Kosher salt (optional) and freshly ground black pepper

1 medium white onion (about 2 cups), trimmed and diced

2 medium carrots (about 1 cup), peeled and diced

1 medium celery stalk, trimmed and diced

4 garlic cloves, diced

2 T tomato paste

1½ cups dry white wine

2½ lbs Roma tomatoes, peeled, seeded, and chopped fine

3 cups chicken stock

Pinch of minced fresh oregano leaves

Pinch of minced fresh thyme leaves

6 or 7 chopped fresh basil leaves

Pinch of red pepper flakes, or to taste

Directions

1. In a 10- or 12-inch sauté pan, heat 3 T of the olive oil. Sauté the ground chicken until lightly browned, breaking up the pieces as they cook. Season lightly with salt and pepper. Remove the chicken with a slotted spoon and drain in a colander. Set aside until needed.

2. In the same sauté pan, heat the remaining 2 T of olive oil. Over medium heat, sauté the onions, carrots, and celery until they just start to color, 6 to 8 minutes. Do not brown. Add the garlic, stir in the tomato paste, and cook a few minutes longer.

3. Deglaze the pan with the wine and cook, stirring occasionally until almost all the liquid has evaporated. Add the tomatoes, cook for 2 or 3 minutes, then pour in the stock and season with the oregano, thyme, and a little salt (optional) and pepper. Cook until the sauce has thickened slightly, about 30 minutes. If the sauce has thickened too much or if you prefer a thinner sauce, add a little more stock. Stir in the chopped basil and the red pepper flakes and adjust the seasoning to taste.

To prepare ahead: Through step 3, this recipe can be prepared one or two days in advance and refrigerated until needed. It also can be frozen for up to four months.

Shepherd's Pie

My daughters Jamie, Lindsay, and Sarah traveled with me when we broadcast *Good Morning America* live from Scotland, England, and Ireland about ten years ago. My most difficult assignment on that trip was finding food that my then three-, seven-, and 10-year-old girls were willing to eat. I've often said that I felt like Columbus discovering America when I stumbled onto Shepherd's Pie. They love the mashed potatoes and ground round, and I love that you can sneak lots of good veggies in too. This is one of those dishes where you can add whatever veggies you have on hand. This recipe serves 4 adult portions.

Ingredients

6 medium red potatoes, peeled and quartered

¼ cup milk

1 T butter

Generous pinch nutmeg

Salt (optional) and pepper

2 T olive oil

2 medium onions, chopped

1 T parsley, finely chopped

1 tsp each dried thyme and sage

1 lb lean ground beef or ground turkey

¼ cup water

2 medium carrots, finely chopped

1½ cups cooked corn (or 1 can corn, drained)

1½ cups cooked peas (or 1 can peas, drained)

2 T all-purpose flour

1 beef bouillon cube

1 tsp granulated sugar

1 tsp ketchup, Dijon mustard, and Worcestshire sauce

Salt (optional) and pepper

Directions

1. *Topping:* Place potatoes in large saucepan of cold, salted (optional) water. Bring to a boil and simmer partially covered for 20 minutes or until very tender. Drain and add milk, butter, nutmeg, and salt (optional) and pepper to taste. Mash potatoes until fluffy. Set aside and keep warm.

2. *Meat filling:* Heat the oil in a large skillet over medium heat. Add onions, parsley, thyme, and sage. Cook for 5 minutes or until onions are soft. Add beef and water and stir frequently to break up meat. Cook until meat is no longer pink. Stir in carrots, corn, and peas. Reduce heat and cook 15 minutes more, mixing well. Stirring continuously, add flour, bouillon cube, sugar, ketchup, mustard, Worcestshire sauce, and salt (optional) and pepper to taste. Cook 5 minutes more and skim fat while cooking.

3. Pour meat filling into a buttered ovenproof casserole dish 9-by-9 or 10-by-10 inches. Spread the potato mixture on top and score top of potatoes with fork.

4. Bake in preheated 350°F oven for 30 to 40 minutes until potatoes are golden brown and meat filling is hot. Serve.

Wolfgang's Wiener Schnitzel

I'm including this "fried" dish because renowned Chef Wolfgang Puck says that in his hometown of Vienna, it's said that a perfectly fried veal schnitzel should be so free of grease that a gentleman could sit down on it and the schnitzel wouldn't even leave a stain on his trousers! That cracks me up, but it also points out that when made properly, this is not a greasy dish.

When buying your veal, be sure that it's no more than ¼ inch thick; if necessary, at home, place each piece of veal between two sheets of plastic wrap and pound with a meat mallet to make the veal even thinner. To give the veal an extra-crispy coating, Wolfgang says to look for the packaged, coarse Japanese-style bread crumbs known as Panko.

Ingredients

Peanut oil for frying

1 cup all-purpose flour

2 eggs, beaten with 2 T cold water

4 cups Panko or fresh, dry white bread crumbs

4 veal scaloppine, 8 oz each

Salt and freshly ground pepper

1 cup whole parsley leaves, rinsed and thoroughly dried

2 lemons, each cut into 4 wedges

Directions

1. In a deep, heavy skillet or saucepan, preheat about 3 inches of oil to 375°F on a deep-frying thermometer.

2. Put the flour, egg mixture, and bread crumbs in each of three large, shallow pie plates, side by side. Season the veal scaloppine on both sides with salt and pepper. One at a time, dredge the scaloppine in flour to coat evenly; dip them on both sides in egg wash; then turn them in the Panko or bread crumbs to coat them evenly. Gently shake off excess crumbs. On a work surface, use a sharp knife to lightly score the breading four times in a crosshatch pattern, to help secure the breading and prevent curling. Carefully slip the scaloppine into the hot oil and deep fry until golden on both sides, about 3 minutes. Remove with a wire skimmer or slotted spoon and transfer to paper towels to drain.

3. As soon as the schnitzels are done frying, put the parsley into the hot oil and fry until dark green and crisp, about 15 to 20 seconds. Remove it with a skimmer or slotted spoon and drain on paper towels. When serving, garnish with parsley and lemon wedges.

Tortilla Chicken Tenders with Easy Corn Salsa

I always found that my kids wouldn't eat a whole chicken breast, but if I bought chicken tenders and cooked them any which way, I was home free! It's always easier to make the breading stick with smaller pieces of chicken, and this recipe from our friends at *Good Housekeeping* magazine uses tortilla chips, which are especially kid friendly and also delicious. They pair the tenders with corn salsa that's a cinch to prepare. Makes 4 adult servings.

Ingredients

2 oz baked tortilla chips

2 tsp chili powder

¼ tsp salt

1 lb chicken tenders

2 ears corn—husks and silk removed (in a pinch, I use frozen corn)

1 jar (11–12 oz) mild salsa

¼ cup loosely packed fresh cilantro leaves, chopped

Lime wedges

Nonstick olive-oil cooking spray

Directions

1. Place tortilla chips in a Ziploc plastic bag. Crush with rolling pin to fine crumbs (you should have about one-half cup tortilla crumbs). On waxed paper, combine crumbs, chili powder, and salt. Set aside.

2. Preheat oven to 450°F. Spray 15½-by-10½-inch jelly roll pan with olive-oil spray. Place chicken tenders in medium bowl and spray with olive oil, tossing to coat well. Roll chicken in tortilla crumbs to coat and place on pan. Spray again.

3. Bake chicken about 10 minutes, or until chicken loses its pink color throughout.

4. Meanwhile, prepare corn salsa: cut corn kernels from cobs; place in small bowl. Stir in salsa and cilantro and blend.

5. Serve chicken with corn salsa and lime wedges.

Turkey Meat Loaf

Whn I was a little girl, my mom often cooked meat loaf. I remember how good it smelled cooking in the oven—and how good it tasted cold in a sandwich a day or two later. That's why I asked the folks in the test kitchen of *Good Housekeeping* magazine to put together a low-fat meat loaf for us using turkey instead of beef. My kids love this version, and I think yours will too.

Ingredients

1 T olive oil	⅓ cup fat-free (skim) milk
2 medium stalks celery, finely chopped	⅓ cup bottled salsa
1 small onion, finely chopped	1 large egg white
2 garlic cloves, finely chopped	½ tsp salt (optional)
¾ tsp ground cumin	½ tsp coarsely ground black pepper
1½ lbs ground turkey breast	¼ cup ketchup
⅓ cup fresh bread crumbs	1 tsp Dijon mustard

Directions

1. In a nonstick 10-inch skillet, heat oil over medium heat. Add celery and onion; cook, stirring often, until vegetables are tender, about 10 minutes. Add garlic and cumin; cook, stirring 30 seconds. Set vegetable mixture aside to cool.

2. Preheat oven to 350°F. In a large bowl, mix vegetable mixture, ground turkey, bread crumbs, milk, salsa, egg white, salt (optional), and pepper with hands until well combined, but not overmixed.

3. In a small bowl, mix ketchup and mustard. Set aside.

4. In a 13-by-9-inch metal baking pan, shape meat mixture into a 9-by-5-inch loaf. Spread ketchup mixture over top of loaf. Bake meat loaf until meat thermometer inserted in center registers 160°F, about an hour (temperature will rise to 165°F upon standing). Let meat loaf stand 10 minutes before removing from pan and slicing. Serve.

Teriyaki Beef and Vegetable Kebabs

One of the secrets to introducing new foods to kids is to make the meal fun. Finger foods, kebabs—whatever it takes to delight and entice them. When I've served my children kebabs, I've often made an assortment; some with beef, some with chicken, some with only vegetables. I've also had success adding a fruit such as pineapple. One suggestion: make the pieces small—kids like little bite-size morsels. Be creative. This recipe makes 8 to 10 adult kebabs.

Note: Be sure to remove skewers when serving to children.

Ingredients

¼ cup light-sodium soy sauce

1–2 cloves garlic, crushed

1 tsp grated fresh ginger

1 tsp lime juice

1 tsp honey

⅛ tsp red pepper flakes

⅛ tsp sesame oil

¾ lb beef tenderloin, fat trimmed and cut into small cubes

1 zucchini cut into ½-inch pieces

1 yellow squash cut into ½-inch pieces

2 Japanese eggplant, cut into ½-inch pieces

1 red pepper, stemmed, seeded, and cut into ½-inch squares

1 Spanish onion, cut into ½-inch wedges

½ lb mushrooms

Directions

1. *Marinade:* In a large bowl, whisk together the soy sauce, garlic, ginger, lime juice, honey pepper flakes, and sesame oil. Transfer 3 tablespoons of this marinade to a medium bowl (reserve balance of marinade) and add beef. Toss to coat. Add zucchini, squash, eggplant, peppers, onions, and mushrooms to the large bowl and toss to coat.

2. Cover and marinate both the meat and vegetables for 30 minutes at room temperature. (Toss once or twice.)

3. Meanwhile, preheat broiler (you can also do these on a grill). Line a broiler pan with aluminum foil and spray with nonstick cooking oil (if you use wooden skewers, make sure to soak in water).

4. Remove the meat and the vegetables from the bowls with slotted spoon and pat dry. Discard marinade.

5. Divide the meat and vegetables equally and thread pieces alternately.

6. Place kebabs in broiler pan, two inches apart. The pan should be four inches from the heat source. Broil 10 to 12 minutes or until the vegetables are tender and the beef is browned (turn once or twice and brush with reserved vegetable marinade).

7. I usually serve over brown rice.

22

Seafood

Chilean Sea Bass Sandwich

At Route 22, a delightful restaurant in Armonk, New York, designed with families and children in mind, this is a regular on the menu. The fish is soft and flaky (the way most kids like it) and the sauce is delicious. Owner Lance Root says it's really easy for moms to make at home, and of course it's packed full of nutrients. Serves 4 (8-oz) adult portions.

Ingredients

2 lbs sea bass (or ask for 4 8-oz fillets)	Tomato slices
Salt (optional) and pepper to taste	Onion slices
4 toasted buns	Pickles
Lettuce	Cajun sauce (See Salmon Burgers)

Directions

1. Fillet two pounds of sea bass into four 8-oz portions.

2. Season with salt and pepper.

3. Grill on barbecue or cook in sauté pan.

4. Serve on toasted bun with lettuce, tomato, onion, and pickle with chips.

5. Use cajun sauce on bun and on side as desired. (See Salmon Burgers for recipe.)

Crab Cakes

If you've got kids in your house, it's a good bet you've got fish sticks in your fridge. Why not try crab cakes as a yummy alternative? I recommend you serve them with sweet corn chowder on page 218. This serves 6 adult portions.

Ingredients

8 oz Maryland lump crabmeat (check for small pieces of shell)

¾ cup fresh bread crumbs

2 tsp Dijon mustard

2 large egg yolks

1 T fresh parsley, chopped

1 tsp kosher salt (optional)

¼ tsp freshly ground pepper

Corn oil for sautéing

Directions

1. Place crabmeat in a bowl. Add bread crumbs and toss lightly to blend. Keep crabmeat in large pieces.

2. Mix mustard, egg yolks, parsley, salt (optional), and pepper together. Pour over crabmeat and bread crumbs. Mix thoroughly—it may seem dry.

3. Form into small 2-inch cakes with your hands.

4. In a medium-size nonstick fry pan, add a small amount of corn oil. When oil is hot, add crab cakes and sauté on both sides until golden and crisp. Serve.

Easy Paella

During my college years, I studied for a while in Mexico City. One of the best parts of that study abroad was, you guessed, the Mexican food. Oh how I love enchiladas, guacamole, and salsa. I can't say that I learned to speak the language fluently, but I did learn to make paella. (A girl's got to have her priorities.) My roommates and I would cook up large vats of it so that we could savor it for days. One of the great things about this dish is that you can vary the ingredients according to what you have available in your kitchen.

Ingredients

3 tsp olive oil

½ lb medium shrimp, peeled and deveined

½ lb sea scallops

½ lb boneless, skinless chicken breast, cut into ½-inch pieces

1 medium onion, chopped (about 1 cup)

2–3 garlic cloves, minced (2 to 3 tsp), or to taste

1 4½-oz can tomatoes, chopped, juice reserved

½ tsp saffron

½ tsp paprika

2 dashes hot sauce or to taste

1 cup medium-grain white rice, preferably arborio

2 cups chicken broth or canned low-sodium chicken broth

4-oz jar sliced pimientos, drained and rinsed

1 cup defrosted frozen peas or corn

½ tsp salt (optional) and pepper to taste

Juice from 2 limes (or 2 T lime juice)

Directions

1. In a large nonstick skillet, heat 1 teaspoon of the oil over moderately high heat. Add the shrimp and sauté for 3 to 4 minutes or until they turn pink.

2. Transfer the shrimp with a slotted spoon to a bowl, and add another teaspoon of the oil to the skillet. Sauté the scallops in the oil for 3 to 4 minutes or until they are very lightly browned.

(continued)

3. Transfer the scallops with the slotted spoon to the bowl. Add the remaining oil to the pan, sauté the chicken for 4 minutes, and transfer it to the bowl.

4. Add the onion and the garlic to the pan, and cook the mixture over low heat for 6 minutes or until the onion is lightly colored.

5. Stir in the tomatoes, saffron, paprika, and hot sauce. Simmer for 3 minutes.

6. Add the rice and stir to coat well.

7. Stir in the broth and bring to a boil. Cover tightly and simmer over low heat for 20 minutes. Add the shrimp, scallops, chicken, pimientos, and peas; cover and cook the paella, stirring occasionally 5 to 10 minutes more, or until the rice is tender. Squeeze limes over dish.

8. Season with salt and pepper to taste.

Pasta Primavera with Shrimp

Most kids like spaghetti, but you don't always have to serve it with sauce or meatballs. Here's a way to make a colorful pasta dish that's loaded with nutrient rich vegetables. I'm adding shrimp, which is low in fat and high in protein, but you can also add chicken to this dish. And of course there are as many variations as you can come up with vegetable combinations. I've used blanched broccoli and cauliflower florets, corn, and thinly sliced zucchini. Serves 6 adults.

Ingredients

½ lb linguini or spaghetti or pasta of choice

2 cups sugar snap peas, trimmed (fresh or frozen)

2 carrots, thinly sliced

½ red bell pepper, thinly sliced

1½ T vegetable oil or butter

1 lb medium shrimp, peeled and deveined

1 garlic clove, minced (about 1 tsp) optional

2 T fresh herbs (i.e. oregano, basil, dill, parsley)

Fresh ground pepper and salt (optional) to taste

1½ cups cherry tomatoes, halved (optional)

1 cup (4 oz) crumbled feta cheese

Directions

1. Cook pasta according to package instructions and drain well.

2. While pasta is cooking, drop peas and carrots into boiling water for 30 seconds, drain, and set aside (these can be dropped in boiling pasta water before it's drained).

3. In a large nonstick skillet, cook red pepper in oil over moderate heat for 5 minutes. Add shrimp, herbs, and garlic, if using, and cook for 3 minutes. Season to taste.

4. Combine pasta, peas, and carrots, and the pepper and shrimp mixture in a large bowl with cherry tomatoes and cheese. Toss well and serve.

Potato-Crusted Snapper

A friend of mine served this delicious fish recipe at her home one evening. When I asked her how she did it, she told me how she had actually planned something much more complicated, but got home late from picking her son up from soccer practice. This was a recipe she said she read in a magazine that had saved her on many occasions when she was flat out of time but had to get dinner on the table. I think we can all relate to that. The instant potato flakes make a light and crispy coating for the fish. (This works great on chicken as well). The recipe serves 4 adult portions.

Ingredients

½ cup low-fat buttermilk

¼ tsp salt (optional)

¼ tsp black pepper

1 clove garlic

¾ cup instant potato flakes (not granules)

2 (6-oz) red snapper or mahimahi fillets

2 T butter or margarine

4 lemon wedges

Directions

1. Combine first four ingredients in a shallow dish. Place potato flakes in another shallow dish. Dip fillets in buttermilk mixture; dredge in potato flakes.

2. Melt butter in a large nonstick skillet over medium heat. Add fish and cook 5 minutes on each side or until golden and fish flakes easily when tested with a fork. You may need to turn several times. Serve with lemon wedges.

Salmon Burgers

Move over cheeseburgers and veggie burgers, because this clever recipe from Route 22 in Armonk, New York, has more nutrients and disease-fighting capability than both of you put together. And, it's easy and tasty! This makes eight 6-ounce adult portions.

Ingredients

1 full side of salmon (2 lb)	6 toasted buns
¼ cup red peppers	Lettuce slices
¼ cup scallions	Tomato slices
¼ cup seafood seasoning	Onion slices
2 whole eggs	Pickles
2 T oregano	Cajun sauce (See next page)

Directions

1. Fillet the full side of salmon. Dice into ½-inch cubes and puree until smooth.

2. Add red peppers, scallions, seafood seasoning, two whole eggs, and oregano with diced salmon and portion out into burgers.

3. Grill on barbecue or cook in sauté pan.

4. Serve on toasted bun with lettuce, tomato, onion, and pickle.

5. Use Cajun Sauce on bun as desired.

Cajun Sauce

Ingredients

1 oz minced garlic

1 quart mayonnaise

1 T Cajun spice

½ cup chives

¾ cup chopped parsley

¼ cup tarragon (medium chop)

½ tsp black pepper

Directions

1. Place first 4 ingredients—minced garlic, mayonnaise, Cajun spice, and chives— in food processor and process.

2. Remove from food processor and place in mixing bowl.

3. Stir in all remaining ingredients.

Yields 5 cups.

Salmon Viareggio

This dish comes from Emilio's, a very popular and charming Italian restaurant in Harrison, New York. I asked owner and chef Sergio Brasesco to craft a salmon dish that would be low on fat, high on flavor, and a short time in the kitchen. Salmon is one of the top three sources of omega-3 fatty acids, which may help prevent heart disease. This recipe serves 2 adult portions.

Ingredients

2 10-oz king salmon fillets

½ cup sundried Gaeta olives

1 leek, julienned

¼ cup whole garlic

¼ cup white wine

Salt (optional) and pepper

2 T extra-virgin olive oil

Directions

1. Rub salmon fillets with salt and pepper, garlic, and a touch of the olive oil.

2. Heat oil over medium heat and sauté the leeks and olives. Season with salt and pepper to taste and remove from heat.

3. Grill salmon fillets for 7 minutes per side.

4. Place salmon fillets in sauté pan with olives and leeks and cook together and add white wine. Let wine cook off.

5. *To plate:* Place leeks on plate first, then salmon, pour olives over the top of the salmon. Serve.

Scallop and Asparagus Stir-Fry

A girlfriend gave me this recipe because she knew I loved scallops. It's very low in fat and filled with lots of colorful veggies. This recipe serves 4 adult portions.

Ingredients

¾ lb asparagus, trimmed and cut diagonally into 2-inch lengths

½ cup reduced-sodium chicken broth

1 T cornstarch

2 tsp soy sauce (or 3 tsp light soy sauce)

12 oz sea scallops

1 cup white mushrooms, trimmed and sliced

1 clove garlic

1 tsp dark sesame oil

1 cup cherry tomato halves

3 small scallions, chopped

Freshly ground black pepper

2 cups cooked rice

Directions

1. Bring one inch of water to boil in saucepan.

2. Add asparagus, cover and cook 3 to 5 minutes (until crisp tender, do not overcook).

3. Drain asparagus and rinse under cold water.

4. In a small bowl, mix chicken broth, cornstarch, and soy sauce until smooth.

5. Meanwhile, heat oil in large nonstick skillet. Place scallops, mushrooms, and garlic in oil and stir-fry over high heat for about 4 minutes, or until scallops are opaque.

6. Stir in cornstarch mixture and cook, stirring until sauce thickens and boils.

7. Add asparagus, cherry tomatoes, and scallions. Season with pepper to taste and stir-fry till heated through.

8. Serve over cooked rice.

Starfish Tuna and Shells

I got this clever recipe from a nutritionist who said it was always a hit with her kids. It's quick and easy and most of us usually have a can of tuna on hand and some sort of pasta. Get yourself some different-shaped cookie-cutters to have fun. This serves 4.

Ingredients

½ (16-oz) box small pasta shells

1 cup crushed cheddar-cheese-flavored crackers

½ tsp seafood-blend seasoning

1 egg, beaten

¼ cup milk

Dash of hot pepper sauce

Dash of Worcestershire sauce

2 cans (6-oz each) tuna packed in water, drained and flaked

¼ cup finely diced red bell pepper

4 tsp olive oil

¼ cup prepared pesto sauce

½ cup grated Parmesan cheese

Salt (optional) and pepper to taste

Directions

1. Prepare pasta shells according to package directions.

2. Stir together crackers, seasoning, egg, milk, hot pepper sauce, and Worcestershire sauce in mixing bowl. Add tuna and bell pepper and mix well.

3. Divide mixture into 6 balls. Flatten each ball into ½-inch-thick circles. Use a 3-inch star-shaped cookie-cutter to shape tuna rounds into starfish shapes.

4. Heat 1 teaspoon of oil in medium skillet over medium-high heat. Place 3 starfish in skillet and cook 2 to 3 minutes, or until bottom is lightly browned. Turn, add another teaspoon of oil to skillet and continue to cook 2 to 3 minutes, or until firm and lightly browned. Repeat process for remaining 3 starfish. Set starfish aside and keep warm.

5. In medium bowl, combine cooked (drained) pasta shells, pesto sauce, and Parmesan cheese. Season to taste with salt (optional) and pepper.

6. Place pasta on serving platter, top with starfish, and serve.

Red Snapper Livornese (Livorno Style)

People make reservations months in advance to dine at the world famous Le Cirque restaurant in New York City, owned by the Maccioni family This wonderful dish comes from *The Maccioni Family Cookbook*. Egi says it's not only one of her husband Sirio's favorites, but that whenever she had a hard time trying to get her kids to eat fish that they would snap up this red snapper. It's amazingly easy and incredibly delicious.

Ingredients

2 lbs red snapper, cleaned and deboned

¼ cup all-purpose flour

3 T olive oil

⅓ cup finely chopped flat-leaf parsley

1 clove garlic, finely chopped

1½ cups peeled and crushed canned tomatoes

¼ cup white wine

Salt (optional) and pepper

Directions

1. Cut the snapper into large pieces. Thoroughly coat the pieces in the flour.

2. Heat the olive oil in a large skillet. Gently fry the snapper pieces over medium heat, just until they begin to turn golden but not entirely cooked, 3 to 5 minutes per side. Remove the fish from the pan and set aside.

3. Add the parsley and garlic to the skillet. Increase heat to medium-high, and cook for 2 minutes. Add the tomatoes and wine and simmer for 10 minutes. Season with salt and pepper to taste.

4. Return the fish to the pan and cover. Reduce the heat and simmer for 10 minutes without disturbing the fish.

5. Carefully transfer the fish pieces to warmed plates and cover with the tomato sauce from the pan. Serve immediately.

23

Veggies and Sides

Baked Acorn Squash

Kids can't resist the sweet flavor of this acorn squash recipe. My mom always used to make it for my brother and me because it was one of our favorites—it's always been a hit with my children as well. Acorn squash is rich in beta-carotene and lutein, vitamins C and B$_6$, and potassium. To cap it off, it's a great source of fiber. This recipe serves 4.

Ingredients

2 acorn squash, halved

1 cup chicken stock

2–3 T unsalted butter

3 T brown sugar

1 tsp ground ginger

¼ tsp nutmeg, fresh or dry

Salt (optional) and fresh ground pepper to taste

Directions

1. Preheat oven to 350°F.

2. Cut each squash in half lengthwise and scrape out seeds and fiber. Place cut side down in a baking dish. Pour the stock over the squash and bake for 20 minutes.

3. Meanwhile, in a small ovenproof bowl, combine the butter, brown sugar, ginger, and nutmeg and place in oven or heat on top of stove for a few minutes to melt butter and sugar.

4. Remove squash from oven and turn over. Fill each squash with 1 tablespoon of butter-sugar mixture. Season with salt (optional) and pepper.

5. Cover dish with wax paper and return to oven for 30 minutes more, till squash is tender. Serve. I sometimes squeeze fresh lemon juice over the top for a fresh burst of flavor.

Steamed Herbed Artichokes

Where I come from in the Sacramento Valley of California, farmers grow many of the fruits and vegetables that serve our nation. Whenever we would make the drive from Sacramento to San Francisco, we would always stop to buy artichokes from the farm stands in what my brother, Jeff, and I called Artichoke Country. There would be rows of the prickly vegetable for as far as the eyes could see. My mom simply cut the ends flat so they would stand in a big pot of water and trimmed off the sharp leaves before simmering them with a little salt, pepper, oil, and parsley. Then she would mix a little curry powder and paprika with mayonnaise for dipping. So I began cooking artichokes for my girls when they were little. This recipe comes from my friends at Da Vinci's restaurant in Greenwich, Connecticut, and serves 4 adult portions.

Ingredients

4 medium-size artichokes	½ cup bread crumbs
½ cup chopped Italian parsley	2 medium-size potatoes
6 scallions	8–10 oz frozen peas
2 cloves garlic	½ cup extra-virgin olive oil
½ cup grated imported Parmesan	

Directions

1. Remove tough outer leaves and pinch inner centers. Cut, remove, and save the stems. Place in cold water with juice of one lemon to prevent discoloration during the preparation of all the ingredients.

2. Chop parsley, garlic, scallions (including green stems), and the reserved artichoke stems. Place all chopped ingredients in mixing bowl with Parmesan and bread crumbs. Toss well.

3. Peel and cube potatoes and place in cooking pan with frozen peas.

4. Gently ease open the leaves of the artichokes and fill equally with all the chopped ingredients.

5. Place open artichokes in a snug-fitting pan with the potatoes and peas and fill with cold water (half of artichokes should be covered with water). Drizzle olive oil on the tops of each artichoke and cover pan with a lid.

6. Bring water to a boil and then reduce heat to a slow simmer. Add small amounts of additional water as it evaporates. Simmer for approximately one hour and fifteen minutes, or until leaves remove easily. Serve.

Broccoli Corn Bread

I've never met a kid who doesn't like corn bread, and this clever recipe turns it into a nutritious treat! The mother of two sets of twins, God bless her, sent this to me upon the birth of my twins. I love that kind of baby gift, and until the twins are old enough to enjoy it, my older girls can indulge and reap the benefits of the phytonutrients abundant in broccoli. This recipe serves 16 yummy, thick, adult slices.

Ingredients

1 10-oz package frozen, chopped broccoli

1 box Jiffy Cornbread Mix

4 eggs

1¼ cup onion, chopped

½ cup cheddar cheese, shredded

Directions

1. Preheat oven to 350°F.

2. Cook broccoli according to package directions and drain.

3. Combine broccoli with remaining ingredients and pour into a 13-by-9-inch baking dish (sprayed with vegetable cooking spray).

4. Bake 25 to 30 minutes or until top is golden brown.

5. Slice and serve.

Broccoli Puff

Broccoli and corn were the only veggies my girls liked when they were little (along with cauliflower, if I'd put cheese on it). One of the reasons they liked broccoli was because I would wrap tinfoil around the stems and make them look like little trees, at least according to my girls. I only cared that I was getting steamed broccoli into my daughters. As it turns out, one of their favorite dishes I make today happens to contain broccoli. Who would've thunk it? So I thought I'd share it with you. It's not my least-fattening dish, but it's good now and then—and easy. I hope it will be a sure hit for you as it has been for me. I'll confess that I sometimes make this really simple dish when company comes, and I always get raves. Even my in-laws will eat this, and they hardly ever eat vegetables. My father-in-law, Donny, jokes that he never met a vegetable he liked. Wait till they read this book; you can bet their new little grandkids will have plenty of fruits and vegetables.

Ingredients

2 10-oz packages chopped broccoli or 2 fresh broccolis, chopped

2 eggs beaten

1 can cream of mushroom soup (low sodium)

1 cup sharp low-fat shredded cheddar cheese

½ cup milk

1 cup mayonnaise

½ cup bread crumbs

Directions

1. Cook the broccoli till soft. Drain and put in a 9-by-9-inch square Pyrex pan (or whatever size you have available).

2. Mix together eggs, soup, cheese, milk, and mayonnaise. Pour over broccoli.

3. Melt 2 tablespoons butter and mix with ½ cup bread crumbs. Sprinkle bread crumb mixture over top of broccoli mixture.

4. Bake at 350°F for 45 minutes. Serve.

Baked Cheesy Potato Gratin

Most kids like anything gooey and cheesy, so this recipe should be a crowd pleaser. You can also add other vegetables, such as chopped broccoli, carrots, parsnips, peas, or all of them. This recipe serves 6 adult portions.

Ingredients

1 lb yellow flesh potatoes, peeled and sliced

1 garlic clove, minced

16 oz fat-free milk

¼ tsp salt (optional)

1 tsp cornstarch

⅛ cup water

⅓ cup Swiss cheese, coarsely grated

½ cup bread crumbs

2 T Parmesan cheese, freshly grated

Directions

1. Preheat oven to 350°F.

2. Combine potatoes, garlic, milk, and salt (optional) in large saucepan, and simmer over medium heat, 8 to 10 minutes, until potatoes are tender.

3. Blend cornstarch with water in a small cup or bowl and stir into potato mixture until slightly thickened.

4. Remove pan from heat and stir in Swiss cheese.

5. Transfer potato mixture to small baking dish.

6. Combine bread crumbs and Parmesan cheese; sprinkle over potatoes.

7. Bake 30 to 40 minutes until the top is brown and mixture is bubbling.

8. Let potatoes rest about 20 minutes before serving.

Twice-Baked Parmesan Potatoes

So what's better than a soft yummy baked potato? You got it, a twice-baked potato! And this version has the added flavor of the Parmesan, while reducing fat by omitting the cheddar cheese, butter, and cream, and substituting low-fat milk. Adding the leeks gives it a mild onion flavor. This recipe serves 4 adult portions.

Ingredients

2 baking potatoes (about ¼ to ½ lbs total)

1 leek, white and pale green part only, finely chopped, rinsed well and patted dry (about ½ cup), or ½ medium onion, finely chopped

1 T olive oil

⅓ cup plus 2 T 1% milk, heated

3 T freshly grated Parmesan

Salt (optional) and pepper to taste

2 tsp finely chopped parsley

Directions

1. Preheat the oven to 425°F.

2. Prick the potatoes a few times with a knife, and bake them in the preheated oven for 1 hour or until tender. Let them cool until they can be handled.

3. While the potatoes are baking, cook the leeks in the oil in a nonstick skillet over moderately low heat for 5 minutes, or until they are softened.

4. Cut the potatoes in half lengthwise and scoop the pulp into a bowl, leaving a ¼-inch-thick shell. Mash the pulp with a fork or a potato masher until it is smooth.

5. Stir into the potatoes: cooked leeks, the milk, 2 tablespoons of the Parmesan, and salt (optional) and pepper to taste.

6. Mound one-quarter of the potato mixture back into the shells. Sprinkle the remaining Parmesan over the top of each mound, and bake the stuffed potatoes in the preheated oven for 10 to 15 minutes or until they are hot. Sprinkle with parsley and serve.

Brown Rice and Asparagus Stir-Fry

At my house I've always found rice (and, of course, pasta) to be the easiest kind of dish to load up with vegetables. And this recipe is like a gold mine, for asparagus provides a hefty amount of the daily folate requirements and is filled with phytochemicals. And the onions are not only cancer fighters, but also defenders of the heart, lowering our cholesterol while boosting the mineral content in our bones to protect us from osteoporosis. And besides that, well, kids just like Chinese food! I also like to make batches of brown rice and keep it in my fridge, which makes this an easy "throw together" on a busy day. This recipe serves 4 adult portions.

Ingredients

2 tsp canola oil

2 cups asparagus trimmed and cut in thirds

1 cup mushrooms, thinly sliced

½ cup onions, chopped

½ cup celery, thinly sliced

2 cups cooked brown rice

2 T light soy sauce

Directions

1. In a large fry pan or wok, heat the oil over medium-high heat. Add asparagus, mushrooms, onions, and celery. Cook, stirring for 5 minutes.

2. Add the cooked brown rice (cook according to package directions) and soy sauce. Cook, stirring for 2 minutes longer. Remove from heat and serve immediately.

Peanut Rice

Y ou can use any kind of rice you have in your cupboard for this recipe. I'm using one of my children's favorites, basmati. But whatever rice you choose, when you add the peanuts, you add heart-healthy fat as well as a tasty crunch. You can also add other vegetables. Serves 4 adult portions.

Ingredients

2¼ cups water

1 cup uncooked white basmati rice

½ tsp salt (optional)

¼ tsp ground turmeric (if not available, combine paprika and cumin)

½ cup dry roasted peanuts

½ cup frozen petite green peas, thawed

Directions

1. Bring water to boil in medium saucepan. Add rice, salt (optional), and turmeric; cover, reduce heat, and simmer 20 minutes or until liquid is absorbed.

2. Remove from heat and stir in peanuts and peas. Mix well and return to heat to bring to serving temperature and serve.

Roasted Vegetables

Roasting or grilling vegetables brings out an enormous amount of flavor. It doesn't get much easier than this folks! Simply brush on a little olive oil to prevent the vegetables from sticking to the pan, and you've got powerful flavor to tantalize your taste buds and powerful nutrients and antioxidants to protect you from disease. Serves 6 adult portions.

Ingredients

2 carrots, peeled and cut into sticks (about 3½ inches)

2 parsnips, peeled and cut into sticks (about 3½ inches)

1 zucchini, cut into sticks (about 3½ inches)

1 red pepper, cut into strips

1 bunch asparagus (about 12 stalks), the tough ends removed and the stalk peeled

Florets from 1 head of broccoli

2 T olive oil

Salt (optional) and pepper to taste

Directions

1. Preheat the oven to 425°F.

2. Arrange all the vegetables in one layer in a large shallow roasting pan, sprinkle them with the oil, and salt (optional) and pepper to taste.

3. Roast vegetables for 35 to 40 minutes until tender. Shake pan every 15 minutes so that vegetables cook evenly.

Rosemary Roasted Sweet Potatoes

How can you lose with a food that is as sweet as sugar and also packed with nutrients? In addition to vitamins, minerals, and fiber, sweet potatoes contain phytochemicals that fight cancer. And as if that's not enough, they also contain immune-boosting carotenoids. Rich in vitamin C, the sweet potato is also loaded with the powerful antioxidant beta-carotene, and yet with all this, it's not loaded with fat. Without getting fancy, you can cook up a succulent sweet potato in minutes for hungry children. This recipe serves 6 adult portions.

Ingredients

2 lbs sweet potatoes, cut in 1½-inch pieces

2 cloves garlic, peeled and finely chopped

1 T chopped fresh rosemary

2 T olive oil

¼ cup toasted pine nuts

2 T chopped parsley

1 T salt (optional) and ¼ tsp ground black pepper

Directions

1. In a roasting pan, combine sweet potatoes, garlic, rosemary, and olive oil; toss to coat well.

2. Roast in 375°F oven for 40 minutes—turn occasionally.

3. Before serving, season with parsley, pine nuts, salt (optional) and pepper.

Quickie sweet potato option: Prick the skin of a whole sweet potato several times and then microwave for 4 to 6 minutes on high power. This is healthy fast food!

Root Mousse

always spend my summers in beautiful Maine at Camp Takajo, a private boys' camp, owned and run by my husband, Jeff. The head chef, Norm Charette, has the task of keeping all the young growing boys and counselors well nourished, so he's always looking for recipes for hearty and healthy kid fare. I gave him the challenge to come up with a recipe for root vegetables that kids would like, and I think this one hits a home run.

Ingredients

½ lb turnips

1 lb carrots

¼ lb potatoes

¼ lb onions

2 T butter

1 T brown sugar

Salt (optional) and pepper to taste

Directions

1. Combine first four ingredients in a large saucepan. Add water and simmer until vegetables are tender.

2. Drain well and transfer to food chopper or processor.

3. Once processed, mix well with butter, add brown sugar, salt (optional) and pepper to taste. Serve.

Creamed Spinach

Okay, I know what you're thinking—creamed! We can't make that! Actually, what we can't do is let vitamin-rich fruits and vegetables pass by our children. Better to pass them yummy low-fat creamed spinach that they'll like and let it become a nutritious family standard. (The same goes for carrots—glaze them with a little brown sugar and butter and kids will gobble them up.) The goal, of course, is to get our kids into the habit of eating vegetables and enjoying them. Then, as they grow older, they'll be more likely to move on to sautéed spinach and steamed broccoli. So that you can get in and out of the kitchen on busy afternoons, I'm going to use frozen chopped spinach in this recipe, but when you have the time, try it with fresh spinach. This serves 6 adult portions.

Ingredients

2 10-oz packages chopped frozen spinach, thawed and drained

4 T butter or margarine

¼ cup all-purpose flour

Salt (optional) and pepper to taste

1 cup whole milk

1 small onion finely diced or 2 T minced onions

½ cup low-fat sour cream

Directions

1. Microwave the spinach 7 minutes to thaw or put the frozen spinach in a saucepan with a little water, and cook over high heat until you can break it apart with a fork. Drain. (If using fresh spinach, wash and remove large stems. Add spinach to boiling water, reduce heat to low and simmer about 10 minutes, stirring occasionally. Drain, refresh, squeeze dry, and chop.)

2. Over medium-low heat, melt 2 tablespoons butter in a saucepan. Stir in flour and salt and pepper until creamed together. Stir in milk, a little at a time. Increase heat to medium. Constantly stir with a whisk until mixture becomes thick and smooth. Remove from heat and set aside.

(continued)

3. Sauté diced or minced onions in the 2 tablespoons of butter until tender. Add spinach (and a little water if needed), lower heat, and cover. Stir several times till almost cooked.

4. When spinach is almost completely cooked, stir in the prepared sauce and add sour cream. Stir well and simmer until completely blended.

Note: My mom used to make creamed spinach like this and she'd sometimes add a dash of sugar or nutmeg. If you're having company and want to give it an interesting kick, you can add minced jalapeño peppers. You can also add ¼ cup of Parmesan cheese for a full-bodied flavor. This recipe can be used for other veggies as well. My kids also liked it when I put this mixture in a baking dish and sprinkled it with bread crumbs (mixed with a touch of melted butter) and baked it for 20 minutes in a 325°F oven.

* Microwave alternative: Put the thawed and drained frozen spinach into a dish and heat in microwave until spinach is hot. Add ¼ cup Parmesan or Asiago cheese.

An emergency shortcut: In a saucepan, stir together one 10-ounce can cream of celery soup (low sodium preferably) with butter and salt and pepper till well mixed, and then add frozen chopped spinach and diced or minced onions. Stir together till piping hot.

Spaghetti Squash

truly believe that spaghetti squash is one of the best fake outs of all time. It's a vegetable no matter how you slice it, but boy does it masquerade as pasta. When cooked it will separate into spaghettilike lengths and have the texture of firm cooked spaghetti. Try this out on your family. It's fast and easy and filled with nutrients, and has only 66 calories in each 8-ounce adult serving.

Ingredients

1 spaghetti squash

Directions

1. Cut squash in half lengthwise, and clean out seeds.

2. Place squash cut side down in a pot with 2 inches of water. Cover and boil for 20 minutes (or in microwave, place squash cut side up in a dish with ¼ cup water, cover with plastic wrap, and cook 10–12 minutes). Remove squash from water and let stand for 10 minutes.

3. Run fork over inside of cooked squash to get spaghettilike strands. Serve hot with butter and Parmesan cheese or with spaghetti sauce.

24

Snacks and Dips

Crispy Zucchini Sticks and Dip

If your kids are like mine, they love fried mozzarella sticks. Well, here's a low-fat alternative to that kid favorite that gives them the health benefits of zucchini. You can also use eggplant or sweet potatoes sliced into rounds. Serves 6 adult portions.

Ingredients

½ cup bottled salsa

¼ cup fat-free sour cream

2 zucchini (about ¾ lb)

⅔ cup seasoned Italian bread crumbs

½ cup yellow cornmeal

2 T grated Parmesan cheese (preferably fresh)

¼ tsp salt (optional)

⅓ cup all-purpose flour

3 large egg whites, lightly beaten

Directions

1. Preheat oven to 450°F. Combine salsa and sour cream; set aside.

2. Cut each zucchini lengthwise into quarters; cut each quarter crosswise into 3 pieces.

3. Combine bread crumbs, cornmeal, cheese, parsley, and salt (optional) in a shallow dish. Dredge zucchini pieces in the flour, then in egg whites, and then in the bread crumb mixture. Repeat process with all remaining zucchini pieces.

4. Place dredged zucchini pieces on a large baking sheet coated with cooking spray. Very lightly spray zucchini pieces and bake for 25 minutes, or until lightly browned and crispy. Carefully turn zucchini halfway through cooking.

5. Serve immediately with salsa dip.

Grilled Cheese Pita Sandwiches

Every kid loves grilled cheese sandwiches; in fact, some kids will eat nothing but grilled cheese sandwiches! I think all of my children went through that stage at one time or another. Well, here's a fun twist on that plain old grilled cheese that packs loads of flavor and important nutrients all inside a pita pocket. This recipe serves 4 adult portions.

Ingredients

4 6-inch plain or whole wheat pitas

4 oz low-fat cheese (cheddar, mozzarella, or Swiss), shredded or coarsely grated

Nonstick vegetable-oil spray

Optional additions: sliced tomatoes, green peppers, and pickles

Sauteed onions and mushrooms

Sliced, pitted olives

Crumbled, cooked turkey bacon

Directions

1. Cut a small slice from one side of each pita to make an opening, and stuff ¼ of the cheese and any optional additions into each opening. (Make sure that any optional addition is wedged in the middle of the cheese, so that the cheese melts evenly and the pita stays crisp.)

2. In a preheated large skillet that has been sprayed with the nonstick vegetable-oil spray, cook the stuffed pitas over moderate heat, covered, for 5 minutes a side or until crispy on both sides.

Edamame-Feta Dip and Toasted Pita Crisps

Long popular in the East, soy foods have only recently found their way into American kitchens. Fresh soybeans are called edamame and can be boiled, popped out of their shell, and eaten warm or cold as a snack. They can also be used in soups, salads, or stir-fries, and they are powerful disease fighters. Another healthy snack idea is this soy-based dip, which can be used with crackers, chips, or toasted pita crisps. Makes 32 crisps.

Ingredients

2 cups frozen shelled edamame

2–3 cloves garlic, peeled

½ cup crumbled feta cheese

2½ T fresh lemon juice

2 T extra-virgin olive oil

¼ tsp salt (optional) to taste

¼ tsp freshly ground pepper

4 whole wheat pitas

Directions

1. Bring a large saucepan of lightly salted water to boil. Add edamame and garlic; return to boil. Reduce heat to medium-low and simmer until edamame are tender, about 5 minutes. Drain, reserving ½ cup of the cooking liquid.

2. Place the edamame (reserve a few to sprinkle on top), garlic, ¼ cup of the cooking liquid, feta cheese, lemon juice, oil, salt (optional) and pepper in a blender or food processor. Puree, scraping down the sides as needed, until completely smooth. Transfer to a serving bowl.

3. Cover with plastic wrap and let it stand for ½ hour at room temperature to allow flavors to blend. Thin with additional cooking liquid to desired consistency, if needed. Serve at room temperature.

4. For toasted pita crisps, preheat the over to 425°F. Cut 4 whole wheat pita breads into 4 triangles each. Separate each triangle at its fold. Arrange them on a baking sheet (rough side up). Spray lightly with olive oil cooking spray, or brush with olive oil. Bake until crisp, 8–10 minutes.

"Holy Guacamole"

This chunky guacamole was given to me by my good friend Elise Silvestri, who I think always makes the best blend around. It can be used as a dip or to complement a meat or chicken recipe. And, of course, in my book, it goes with just about any Mexican dish you can come up with. It's filled with fiber, folate, potassium, and other nutrients that can reduce the risk of heart disease and cancer. Obviously, avocados can add up your calorie count, so don't go hog wild!

Ingredients

1 large tomato, seeded and chopped into small pieces

1 clove garlic, finely chopped

½ red onion, finely chopped

½ red bell pepper, seeded and finely chopped

4–5 cilantro branches, chopped, to taste

1 lime

3 soft avocados, peeled and pitted

Tabasco sauce, to taste

Directions

1. Mix first five ingredients. Add the juice of half a lime to the mixture.

2. Mash the avocados with a fork, one by one. Add salt to taste (optional) and the balance of lime juice.

3. Mix avocados with chopped veggies and add Tabasco.

4. If not serving immediately, leave the avocado pits in the bowl to preserve the dip.

5. Serve with fresh veggies or baked tortilla chips.

Quick and Easy Hummus

This delicious chickpea dip, with its Mediterranean influence, is packed full of protein and fiber. Serve it with pita wedges or sesame crackers, carrot sticks, celery, or your child's favorite veggie. My girls love it, and I'm sure your kids will, too. Recipe makes 2 cups.

Ingredients

1 15-oz can chickpeas (garbanzo beans)

3 T sesame tahini (sesame seed butter)

Juice of 1 lemon

2 cloves garlic, crushed

Celery, carrot sticks, baked tortilla chips, or pita wedges

Directions

1. Drain chickpeas, reserve liquid.

2. Place chickpeas in blender or food processor with ¼ cup of reserved liquid. Add tahini, lemon juice, and garlic. Blend until smooth.

3. Serve with celery, carrot sticks, chips, or pita wedges.

Yogurt-Cucumber Dip (Raita)

I remember the first time I took my daughters to an Indian restaurant. I wasn't sure how they would fare with the new flavors and textures. But in fact they loved the potato-filled bread, the tandoori-cooked chicken, the rice with nuts and vegetables, and the yogurt-cucumber dip called raita. I knew I could serve this as a snack at home with pita bread wedges or chips or as an accompaniment for chicken or lamb. It's basically a light and tangy cucumber-yogurt sauce. This recipe makes 2 cups.

Ingredients

1½ cups peeled, seeded, and finely chopped cucumbers

1½ cups plain nonfat yogurt

½ tsp salt (optional)

1 T finely chopped fresh mint (or 1 tsp dried)

½ tsp paprika

Directions

1. In a bowl, stir together the cucumber, yogurt, and salt. If you like a kick to it, you can add a pinch of freshly ground black pepper and a pinch of cayenne. This can be served immediately or refrigerated for 1 to 2 hours.

2. Sprinkle with mint and paprika and serve.

Bruschetta/Crostini

Ingredients

Olive- or vegetable-oil spray

1 thin baguette or loaf of Italian bread, cut crosswise into ⅓-inch-thick slices

Tomato Topping

½ lb tomatoes (about 2 medium), seeded and chopped

½ garlic clove, minced (about ½ tsp) (optional)

1 tsp extra-virgin olive oil

1½ T shredded fresh basil

Salt (optional) and pepper to taste

Directions

Bruschetta: Prepare a grill or heat a grill pan and spray it with the nonstick olive-oil spray. Arrange the bread on the grill 4 inches from the coals (or right on the grill pan if using) and grill it for about 2 minutes a side or until it is lightly browned.

Crostini: Arrange bread in one layer on a baking sheet and toast it in a preheated 400°F oven or toaster oven for 10 minutes.

In a bowl, stir together all tomato topping ingredients, and add salt and pepper to taste. Mound a heaping teaspoon on top of each slice.

Mango Salsa

My friends at the *Good Housekeeping* test kitchen created this new and different salsa to use for a tasty dip or with salmon steaks. The combination of mango and kiwifruit gives this salsa its sweet and tangy flavor. You can also try substituting chopped pitted fresh cherries and a diced yellow pepper for the mango and kiwi. Makes about 4 cups.

Ingredients

2 ripe medium mangoes, peeled and coarsely chopped

2 medium kiwifruit, peeled and coarsely chopped

3 T seasoned rice vinegar

1 T grated peeled fresh ginger

1 T minced fresh cilantro leaves

Directions

1. In a medium-size bowl, combine mangoes, kiwifruit, rice vinegar, ginger, and cilantro.

2. If not serving immediately, cover and refrigerate.

25

Desserts

Blueberry Cobbler

Blueberries are packed full of super cancer-fighting antioxidants. They're yummy when eaten fresh, and of course, we often see them in muffins and pancakes. But this recipe lets the blueberry be the star! Serves 6 adult portions.

Ingredients

Fruit filling

½ cup sugar

2 T cornstarch

4 cups fresh or frozen blueberries

1 tsp fresh lemon juice

Biscuit topping

½ cup all-purpose flour

1 T + 1 tsp sugar

1½ tsp baking powder

4½ oz reduced-fat milk

3 T + 1 tsp vegetable oil

Directions

1. Preheat over to 400°F.

2. *To make fruit filling:* Mix together sugar and cornstarch in a large saucepan, and then stir in blueberries and lemon juice. Cook over medium-high heat until mixture thickens and boils, stirring often. Continue to stir while mixture boils for 1 minute. Pour into a small, ungreased baking dish. Cover to keep hot.

3. *To make biscuit topping:* In a medium bowl, whisk together the flour, sugar, and baking powder. Add the milk and oil, and stir with a wooden spoon until dough forms. Drop the dough onto the top of the fruit mixture in 6 mounds.

4. Bake for 25 to 30 minutes, or until biscuit topping is golden brown. Serve warm.

Bread Pudding

This is a delicious and nutritious dessert that could also double as breakfast! For variation and for added nutrients and fiber, I recommend you top it with fresh strawberries or raspberries or applesauce.

Ingredients

6 cups cubed bread, white, whole wheat (preferably), raisin cinnamon—whatever you have

1½ cups freshly grated apple, or ½ cup raisins (or craisins)

½ cup chopped walnuts, or other nuts (optional)

3 cups milk

3 eggs

½ cup brown sugar

1 tsp cinnamon

¼ tsp nutmeg

2 tsp vanilla extract

¼ tsp salt (optional)

1 T lemon juice

Directions

1. In a 9-by-13-inch baking pan, distribute the cubed bread, grated apple (or raisins/craisins), and the chopped nuts.

2. In a bowl, beat together the milk, eggs, brown sugar, cinnamon, nutmeg, vanilla, salt (optional), and lemon juice.

3. Pour the milk/egg mixture over the bread mixture. Let it soak a few minutes before baking.

4. Bake at 350°F for 40 to 45 minutes, or until the bread pudding is lightly browned and a knife inserted in the center comes out clean.

Carrot Cake

Bugs Bunny was smarter than we all give him credit for. Carrots, his favorite, are packed with phyto-nutrients, which may help protect us from cancer, stroke, and loss of eyesight. This is a sweet, delicious, and nutritious recipe that is quick and easy to make and will delight your children.

Ingredients

¼ cup margarine, softened (non-transfat margarine)

½ cup sugar

2 eggs

¼ cup low-fat milk

½ tsp vanilla extract

¾ cup shredded carrots (about 2)

1 cup flour

1 tsp baking powder

¼ tsp cinnamon

¼ tsp nutmeg

1 T confectioners' sugar (optional)

Vegetable-oil cooking spray

Directions

1. Preheat oven to 350°F.

2. Blend margarine and sugar until well blended.

3. Add egg, milk, vanilla, and carrots.

4. In a small bowl, combine flour, baking powder, cinnamon, and nutmeg. Add this to carrot mixture and blend well.

5. Spray an 8-by-8-inch pan with vegetable-oil cooking spray and pour the batter into the pan.

6. Bake for approximately 30 minutes, until center of cake springs back easily when touched.

7. Cool. Sprinkle with confectioners' sugar, if desired. Serve.

Chocolate Pudding

When I was a little girl, my favorite dessert was chocolate pudding, so I couldn't wait to make it for my daughters. This is a healthier version than the one my mom made for my brother and me, but my children loved it just the same. I still get a craving every now and then for a rich, smooth, creamy pudding, and this recipe will delight the child in all of us. Makes 6 adult servings.

Ingredients

2 tablespoons sugar

¼ cup cocoa

3 T cornstarch

Pinch of salt (optional)

1½ cups evaporated skim milk

½ cup skim milk

¼ cup light or dark corn syrup

1 large egg

1 oz bittersweet (or semisweet) chocolate, chopped

Directions

1. In a saucepan, whisk together the sugar, cocoa, cornstarch, and salt (optional). Whisk in the milks and the corn syrup, and bring the mixture to a boil over moderately high heat, whisking constantly. Boil the mixture for 1 minute, then remove it from the heat.

2. In a bowl, beat the egg lightly and whisk in 2 tablespoons of the hot chocolate mixture. Add the egg mixture to the saucepan, and cook the pudding over moderate heat for 1 minute, whisking. Stir in the bittersweet chocolate, and transfer the pudding to a bowl.

3. Cover the surface directly with plastic wrap. Let it cool and chill well before serving.

Mexican Flan

When I was in my teens, I lived in Mexico for three years, where I went to college. My favorite restaurant had a delicious dessert called flan. When my girls Jamie, Lindsay, and Sarah were quite young, I introduced them to Mexican food. They too loved flan as a dessert. Try this recipe on your family. It has lots of calcium, magnesium, and riboflavin.

Ingredients

⅓ cup sugar

1 12-oz can skim or low-fat evaporated milk

1 14-oz can sweetened condensed milk

½ cup milk

5 eggs

2 tsp cornstarch

2 tsp vanilla

Directions

1. Preheat oven to 350°F.

2. Heat sugar in a saucepan over medium heat, shaking it occasionally. The sugar will begin to turn to syrup; keep shaking until it has become golden brown.

3. Remove syrup from heat and pour into an 8-inch-square baking dish.

4. Blend remaining ingredients in food processor or blender, first on low, then on high heat until well mixed.

5. Pour blended egg mixture into baking dish. Cover with foil, making sure foil does not touch the mixture. Put into a larger baking dish. Pour 1 inch of hot water into outer dish.

6. Bake for 50 to 60 minutes until a knife inserted into the middle comes out clean.

7. Remove carefully and set out to cool.

8. Place a serving platter on top of the flan dish and turn upside down, so that flan comes out on the platter with the syrup side up. Serve.

Peach Crisp

We sometimes forget that fresh fruit makes a tasty and wonderfully nourishing dessert. Every survey tells us the same sad story—Americans simply don't eat enough fruit. So we obviously need some exciting dishes to entice us, and I think this one meets that challenge.

Ingredients

3 cups sliced fresh, frozen, or canned (drained) peaches

½ cup brown sugar, packed

½ cup flour

½ cup oatmeal

1½ tsp cinnamon

¼ cup soft butter (½ stick)

Directions

1. Put 3 cups of peaches in the bottom of a 10-by-6- or 8-by-8-inch baking pan.

2. In a large bowl, mix together the brown sugar, flour, oatmeal, and cinnamon. Then, using an electric mixer, cut the soft butter evenly into the dry ingredients.

3. Sprinkle the mixture evenly over the fruit. If you prefer more topping, you can make two thin layers of fruit with two layers of topping.

4. Bake at 375°F around 40 to 45 minutes, or until the top is slightly browned. The fruit should feel tender when you test with a toothpick.

Variation: You can use an equal amount of apples (peeled or unpeeled), pears (cored and sliced), blueberries, blackberries, or fresh plums (pitted and sliced). To cut down on your time in the kitchen, consider doubling or tripling the recipe and refrigerating it in a glass container so that when you make another crisp, all you have to do is prepare the fruit!

Pumpkin Pudding

I think it's such a shame that Thanksgiving only comes once a year because it's certainly one of my favorite meals, especially the pumpkin pie! A terrific friend, who lived with us for many years to help with the children, found this recipe for all of us pumpkin lovers. It's not as elaborate as a Thanksgiving meal, in fact, it's incredibly quick and easy, and has calcium and vitamin A. This recipe serves 6 adult portions.

Ingredients

15-oz can pumpkin	¾ tsp baking powder
2 eggs	½ tsp baking soda
12-oz can evaporated skim milk	½ tsp cinnamon
1 cup sugar	½ tsp ginger
2 tsp lemon juice	½ tsp nutmeg
¾ cup flour	

Directions

1. Preheat oven to 350°F and lightly oil a 3-quart casserole or soufflé dish.

2. In a large bowl, mix together pumpkin and eggs until smooth. Then whisk in milk and lemon juice.

3. Measure all dry ingredients and add to pumpkin mixture. Blend thoroughly.

4. Pour mixture into prepared casserole and bake for 40 to 50 minutes until set.

5. Serve warm with vanilla frozen yogurt.

Very Berry Ambrosia

You can make ambrosia with many different fresh fruit combinations. It's not only colorful but also boosts the immune system and helps to lower cholesterol levels, and makes a beautiful and delicious dessert.

Ingredients

2 cups orange sections	8-oz can pineapple chunks
2 cups strawberries (halved if large)	½ cup flaked coconut
2 cups blackberries	2 T honey
2 cups raspberries	

Directions

1. Arrange half of the orange sections in a glass bowl. Top with half of the strawberries, blackberries, raspberries, pineapple chunks, and coconut. Repeat layers.

2. Drizzle with honey and sprinkle with remaining coconut.

3. Cover and chill until ready to serve.

Index